I0489567

Health

is

Wealth

and it is Tax-Free

Health
is
Wealth
and it is Tax-Free

CA. Dr. Vishnu Bharath Alampalli

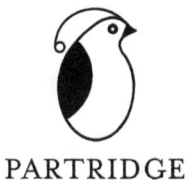

PARTRIDGE

Copyright © 2016 by CA. Dr. Vishnu Bharath Alampalli.

ISBN:	Hardcover	978-1-4828-7153-1
	Softcover	978-1-4828-7152-4
	eBook	978-1-4828-7151-7

All rights reserved. No part of this book may be used or reproduced by any means, graphic, electronic, or mechanical, including photocopying, recording, taping or by any information storage retrieval system without the written permission of the author except in the case of brief quotations embodied in critical articles and reviews.

Because of the dynamic nature of the Internet, any web addresses or links contained in this book may have changed since publication and may no longer be valid. The views expressed in this work are solely those of the author and do not necessarily reflect the views of the publisher, and the publisher hereby disclaims any responsibility for them.

Print information available on the last page.

To order additional copies of this book, contact
Partridge India
000 800 10062 62
orders.india@partridgepublishing.com

www.partridgepublishing.com/india

INDEX

PREFACE

"HEALTH IS WEALTH" AND IT IS TAX FREE!

In this world, everything is taxed and fortunately - Health and Smile/Laughter is not taxed yet anywhere in the Globe and make best use of it Before it is Taxed! I am sure one will agree that the words of wisdom and experience will never go wrong. Health is so very important in everybody's life and one can work effectively only if health is sound. Possessing everything and not keeping good health will be disaster and every other thing become useless.

In normal course, one neglects health and only concentrates on everything, specially earning, and only realizes how health is important, when health is deteriorated. Health cannot be bought or captured and it is only a care has to be taken. It is better to sweat it out, burn the extra calories and keep fit.

Our forefathers have invented Yoga and many such activities to keep one fit. I am making an attempt in this book to consolidate all interesting things about the health for useful reading so that it could be digested to improve health by all means, possible. I have been conferred honorary doctorate for social service and, therefore, my prefix need not be mistaken as qualified medical doctor.

I find that we follow certain things, without knowing. Intention is to know fully and follow correctly for keeping good health to enjoy the life. We live to eat or we eat to live but should have good health for effective and useful living. That is why our elders have correctly expressed that health is your first wealth and everything else is secondary and nothing is so very important than health.

I dedicate this book of mine to my beloved mother who did not enjoy a good health and who kept on saying and cautioning others to take care of good health.

CA Dr. Vishnu Bharath Alampalli

FOREWORD

"Prevention is better than cure". I am indeed happy that my good friend Dr A.S. Vishnu Bharath, Chartered Accountant, has come out with a novel idea of bringing a booklet about the tips of sound health. He has covered all useful tips on health. I have glanced it and found very useful and it reminds me that "Prevention is better than cure".

I strongly advise to keep good health by trimming oneself by all means. It is very true that health is your first and valued wealth.

Dr Vivek Jawali
Heart Surgeon
FORTIS – Bengaluru, India

HUMAN LIFE IS VERY PRECIOUS

Human life is very very precious. After many births, one is believed to be born as human. Each and every day is Lord's gift. Life is like a flower that blooms, gives fragrance and fades away. Life is also like a bubble, it may burst any moment if health is not properly taken care off. The very purpose itself is defeated, if not enjoyed. So, enjoy every moment of life with a smile on face. Smile and smile; one has to go miles and miles and, therefore, maintain good health.

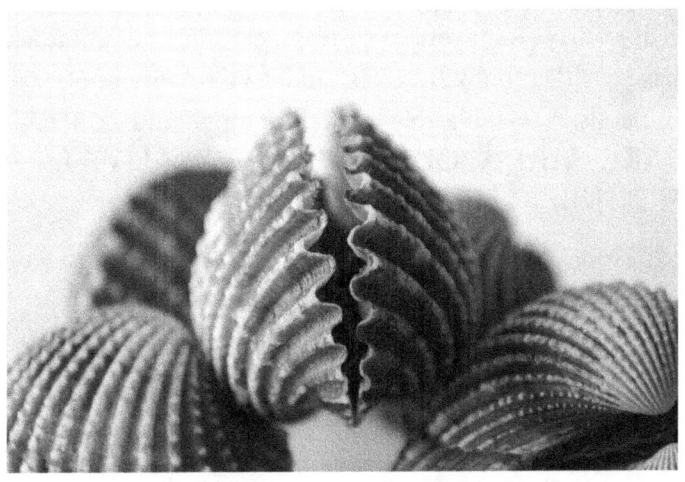

https://pixabay.com/en/shells-scallops-mollusk-marine-166894/

Health is status of physical, mental and social wellbeing. Good health enables to enjoy life and have the opportunity and enthusiasm to achieve the goals. In order to maintain good health one should have basic knowledge about the human body and its functions.

All parts of the body must work together properly to have good health. He/she alone have strength and energy to enjoy life, withstand stress, face any consequences and overcome all types of situations and circumstances. Proper nutrition, exercise, rest, sleep, cleanliness and medical care are all most essential parts of health. A balanced diet provides all the food substances needed by the body for healthy growth and development. The food consists of carbohydrates, fats, proteins, vitamins and minerals. Food and water are most essential. The balanced diet should have wide variety of foods, fluids and vegetables, meat, poultry, fish, etc. Dairy products and nuts are rich sources of proteins. Bread, cereals and potatoes have rich carbohydrates in addition to vitamins and minerals. Vegetables have good vitamins and minerals. TAKE CARE ABOUT YOUR HEALTH LIVE LIFE WITHOUT LIMITS!

TIPS FOR GOOD HEALTH

Health is so very important, one realize only when there is set back in health. Normally it is human tendency to over work even at the cost of Health to acquire the wealth. But one should know that the same Wealth has to be spent back to regain health and some time it may be more than the wealth acquired and hence there is no point to have wealth without good health. As for as possible we have to correct ourselves in day to day work, normally the following are done without knowing it's bad effect on our body and organs:

1) Over drink Coffee.
2) Drinking cool water along with tablets.
3) Using mobile for long conversations.
4) Sufficient water is not drunk during the day time.
5) Taking the water immediately after the heavy food.
6) Taking heavy meal after the sunset.
7) Sleep late in the night and get up late in the morning.

8) **Just lie down immediately after taking medicine.**

9) **Use the mobile phone until the charge is over.**

10) **Taking medicine in empty stomach.**

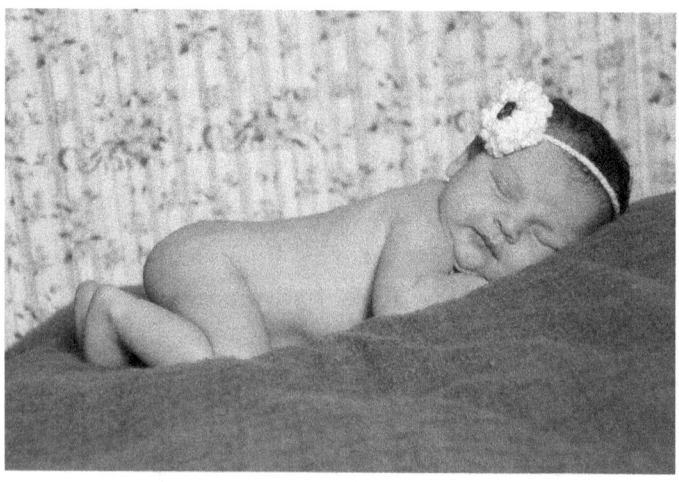

https://pixabay.com/en/baby-child-newborn-health-808371/

The right food maintains health while the wrong food produce disease.

- Eat only when you are hungry, never over eat.
- In all things balance and moderation is the key note.
- Diseases of old age are not due to old age, but are due to wrong living.
- Your personality is the product of your food habits.

- Fight fatigue with diet.
- Give rest to the stomach between two meals at least 4 to 5 hours.
- God provided the Healing power in each body to maintain health.

Tough times are like physical exercise, you may not like it while you are doing it but tomorrow you will be stronger because of it.

Whenever we do something positive in life even if no one is watching, we rise a little bit in our own eyes. Think good, be good, do good.

MIND is not a dustbin to keep anger, hatred and jealousy. But it's a TREASURE box to keep love, happiness and sweet memories.

One in three cases of Cancer is linked to poor eating habits.

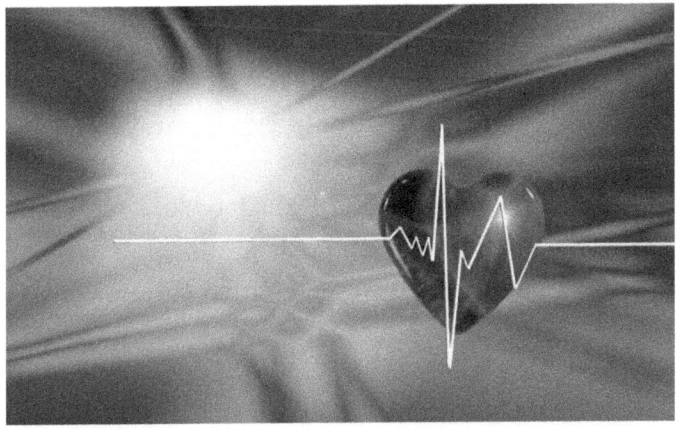

https://pixabay.com/en/heart-curve-bless-you-pulse-66888/

- A living body is maintained by proper breathing, drinking &eating.
- Relax and have a positive and alert mind.
- Do not eat beyond your needs.
- He who eats once is yogi who eats twice is Bogi, who eats thrice a Rogi and who eats four times a day is one whom death welcomes.
- Do not eat when under emotional stress or when extremely fatigue.
- Exercise keeps health in a perfect level.
- Do not swallow until the food has been thoroughly masticated. Food is medicine.
- Make it a practice to eat slowly and chew your food thoroughly.
- Drink the solid and eat the liquid. It is a good policy not to take liquids with meals.
- Drink the water half an hour before meals and two hours after meals.
- Always select simple dishes make sure that your meals are prepared in a Natural way as possible.
- Do not eat until the previous meal has been digested.
- The person lives on half the food he eats and the doctor lives on the other half.
- The best drinks are pure water, fruit juices and vegetables soups.
- Occasional fast on fruit juices can do wonders for your Health.
- Do not eat just for eating sake, eat for Health.
- A healthy digestion is the key to a Happy Life.

- Garlic made into syrup with honey for cough & Asthma.
- To take food do not see the clock for time, your stomach is the clock.
- Miss your meal when you don't feel hungry.
- He who over eats will have all ailments.
- Be sure to thoroughly masticate your food.
- All living power is within your body.
- There are no curative powers in drugs, medicines, herbs anything else outside your own body.
- Do not eat when you are made, bad, sad, but eat when you are glad.
- Nature cure assists people to get well by removing causes of
- Diseases and providing most favorable conditions.
- As stomach has no teeth chew and masticate your food in your mouth only.
- The average adult's weight is made up of about two per cent Calcium.
- Do not feel sorry for yourself when giving up foods not conducive to / good health
- People who eat breakfast are less likely to overeat later in the day.
- If milk is removed from the diet, it can lead to an inadequate intake of calcium
- Avoid alcohol @ least for 5-6 hr before sleep, instead take milk for a better sleep
- If you start your morning with the 10 min of exercise, you will boost your metabolism by 15%

- Drink 1.5-2 ltr of water a day 2 hydrate body, reduce fatigue and help brain work
- For every minute you are angry, you lose sixty seconds of happiness!
- Our body is a machine for living. It is organized for that, it is its nature. Let life go on in it unhindered and let it defend itself, it will do more than if you paralyze it by encumbering it with remedies.

NATURE CURE IS A WAY OF LIFE

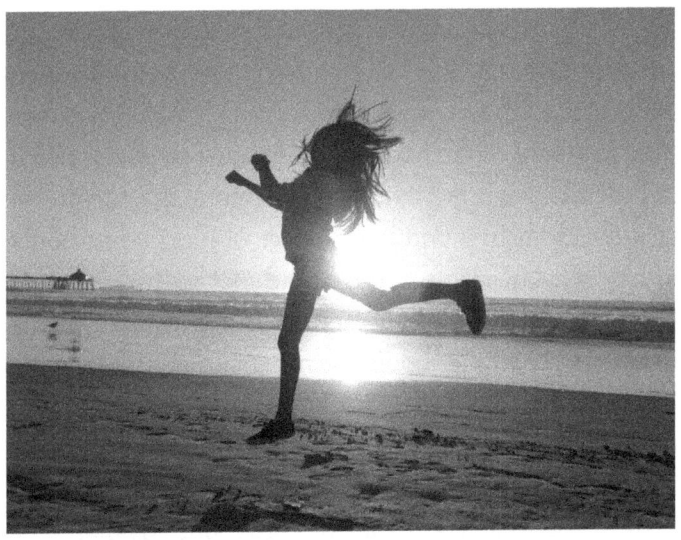

https://pixabay.com/en/girl-jump-happy-active-activity-324688/

"A sound mind in a sound body" - the more fit one's heart is, the more one's brain seems to benefit. This old adage underlines the importance of a healthy body. A healthy body is obtained by maintaining a good diet and good exercise to keep the body going. A good exercise consists of vigorous exercises or yoga and other such things. To keep the mind clean we should always have a positive thinking and honest attitude in life. Health is not something that can be purchased in a bottle from a drug store, but it is a condition built over the years from within by our own vital processes through conscientious efforts and self-control or will power. It is a source of happiness as it helps create an atmosphere of amiable interaction with our near and dear ones.

Unfortunately, in the minds of many people, including doctors, nature cure not stand for any definite school or scientific system of medicine and a number of unqualified persons practicing nature cure are simply defaming. The time has come when nature cure should be standardized; in order to give it its rightful place among the sciences of healing. A healthy body is a source of pleasure not only to one self but also to others who look at it. A healthy person can think normally and act instantly in any given situation. A sound body means a healthy body, free from diseases and it does not bulky body. A sound mind means a mind capable of good, positive and free thinking mind. Thus, to possess a healthy body and mind with naturopathy is a great social and economic advantage.

HOW TO IMPROVE HEALTH BY FASTING

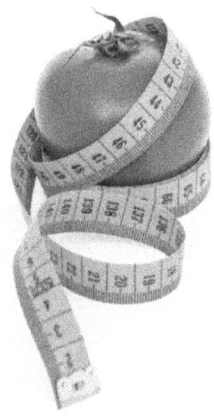

https://pixabay.com/en/tape-tomato-diet-loss-weight-403591/

Excessive food intake, current way of life, luxuries and lack of exercise have been the leading cause for health complications. All religions recognize and recommend fasting and it is proved even in the science that frequent fasting is good for health. This is because fasting tends to give rest to all organs, overhaul the systems, and eventually eliminate toxins from the body. In other words, regular fasting acts like cleansing process. So, by fasting twice a month, one gets not only health benefits but also spiritual benefits. It may be difficult to begun fasting, but gradual reduction and determination of mind alone can help regular fasting. Animals and birds are not as brainy as humans, look at the animals they do not take any intake when they are ill and they get better and this undoubtedly indicate fasting is the best healer for illness. Fasting is therefore quickest, cheapest, simplest and proved way of healing most type of illness. The food taken is always excessive, even 25% of the normal intake is just sufficient for body to get energy required and the excess intake naturally harms the various organs of human body. The major organs of human body are stomach, intestines, kidney, pancreas, lungs etc., which are continuously working and by fasting they not only get rest but also acts as mechanism of cleaning, overhauling and purifying the system.

In short, fasting is a real cleansing device-an overhauling and purifying process. Periodical fasting is very essential to keep the body healthy, but fasting for longer periods should be undertaken only under the guidance of an expert/naturopath.

Listening is an art, In the current readymade world we always listen the vehicle sound, vehicle honking sound, gossip, television, FM radios or few crazy meaningless song. Do we get any kind of energy by listening to these sounds? we never listen to ourselves, we keep the alarm in one time and wake up at different time, we promise ourselves that today I will start jogging, cycling, have right diet, start studying something, car service, insurance renewal, health checkup etc. do you know one thing "All the problems in our life is created by ourselves by not listening to our own soul". Listen, listen and keep listening before reacting to anything and give yourself an appointment on daily basis to listen to all the good deeds or listen the AUM the first sound in the universe which will give you abundant energy.

90% OF FOOD INTAKE VERSUS 10% ANALYSIS:

90% of worries are due to 10% of over eating.

90% of your energy is derived from 10% of food eaten.

90% of tension is created by 10% of carelessness

90% of food eaten is junk – only 10% gives all energy needed.

90% of illness could be cured naturally – only 10% needs medication.

90% of rich have health problems – 10% only enjoy good health.

90% of exercises, if not done properly it is waste – only 10% helps out.

90% of fibrous food and 10% of tasty food is OK.

90% of hunger could be managed by 10% of food intake.

90% of diseases of old age are due to 10% of carelessness.

HEALTH OF MIND

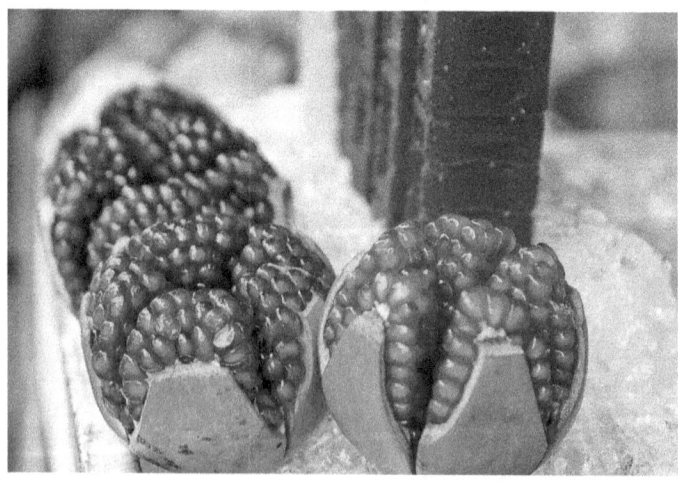

https://pixabay.com/en/pomegranate-juice-fruit-fresh-food-463376/

- The trouble with always trying to preserve the health of the body is that it is so difficult to do without destroying the health of the mind.
- Take care of your body. It's the only place you have to live."
- The more severe the pain or illness, the more severe will be the necessary changes. These may involve breaking bad habits, or acquiring some new and better ones.

- To insure good health: eat lightly, breathe deeply, live moderately, cultivate cheerfulness, and maintain an interest in life.
- Cheerfulness is the best promoter of health, and is as friendly to the mind as to the body.
- The preservation of health is a duty. Few seem conscious that there is such a thing as physical morality.
- Happiness is nothing more than good health and a bad memory.
- People who are always taking care of their health are like misers who are hoarding a treasure which they have never spirit enough to enjoy.
- A healthy breakfast should include complex carbohydrates such as whole grain breads, oatmeal, or broken wheat porridge.
- Do not lick your chapped lips as saliva is not a moisturizer. It will only dry your lips much more.
- Avoid unhealthy accompaniments and garnishing. A healthy grilled sandwich becomes a fatty meal if eaten with Frenchfries.
- Saturated fat weaken your immune system as they induce a state of low-grade inflammation in your body & decrease its ability to fight infections.
- Consuming yoghurt or curd can enhance your immunity because it contains good bacteria that stimulate the immune.

- You can have a protein rich but low fat diet by consuming fish, seafood, egg whites, pulses, beans, and soy products.

- Avoid using steroid based over-the-counter medicines for fungal infections as they can lower skin's immunity and make infection worse.

- To get a good amount of vitamin C add guavas, papayas, oranges, and melon to your diet.

- To prevent aches and pains after long hours of computer use, take periodic breaks to do stretch exercises at your desk.

- Make fists with both hands, and then relax. This maneuver gets flowing to your hand muscles and can relieve pain caused by typing.

- If you have heat rash, do not use a towel after a shower and allow your body to air dry. The rash will disappear faster.

- Seafood such as oysters, sardines, clams, crab and fish produce a mood enhancing effect by supplying plenty of selenium.

- Avoid regular consumption of high salt items such as pickles and ketchups as excess sodium is a risk factor for high blood pressure.

- Watch out for these words while ordering food: rich gravy, cheese or cream sauce, coconut milk, Au gratin. They indicate "very fatty".

- Sliced cucumber with some salt and pepper is the perfect summer snack as it replenishes both water and electrolytes.

- Instead of cold coffee, try iced tea this summer. It's much lower in calories and also has antioxidant properties.
- Avoid a heavy meal after 8:00 pm. It protects you against indigestion, heartburn and weight gain.
- Dark chocolate is a mood booster as it has caffeine and the bromine that have a mood enhancing effect.
- Chuck carbonated beverages this summer and try lower calorie options such as lemonade or tender coconut water.
- Start dinner with a mixed green salad. It help reduce your appetite for caloric foods will automatically add veggies to your meal.
- Do eat when you are hungry. Try to substitute healthier snacks.
- If you often feel sleepy despite spending eight hours or more in bed make sure you do not have sleep apnea that interrupts your sleep.
- Looking out for ways to increase your calcium intake? Add some tofu to your diet. Half cup can give you almost 250mg calcium.
- Avoid too much white bread, potatoes, white rice, and pastries as they quickly boost blood sugar and may raise risk of type 2 diabetes.
- Want to add whole-grains to your diet and wondering what they are? Try oatmeal, brown rice, popcorn, barley and whole-wheat flour.

- When buying margarine and spreads, lookout for those fortified with plant sterols as they help lower LDL cholesterol.
- Having a handful of almonds a day may lower LDL ("bad") cholesterol and reduce your risk of heart disease, heart attack, and diabetes.

OBSERVE ABSOLUTE SILENCE ONCE A MONTH

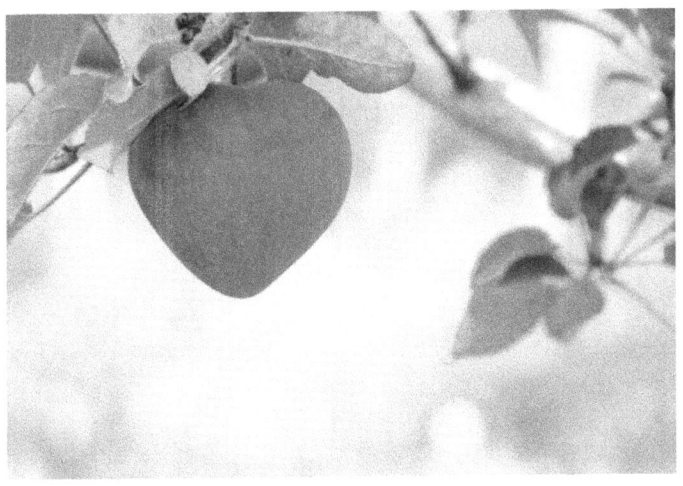

https://pixabay.com/en/apple-love-heart-570965/

"Never raise your voice, just improve the quality of your arguments". As cold water and warm iron take away the wrinkles of clothes, a cool mind and warm heart takes out the worries of life.

Silence brings happiness, peace, rest to throat, time to think, have time for yourself and many more. Absolute silence for the full day has proved to improve the health in every respect. Kind words can be short and easy to speak but their echoes are truly endless.'

Finally, "Heart is the only machine that works without any repair for years" Always keep it happy, whether it is yours or "others".

When you are in the light, everything will follow you when you are in the dark, even your own shadow does not follow you. So, always be in the light.

No and yes are two shortest answers which need a long thought. Most of the things we miss in life only because of saying no too early or yes too late.

HOW MUCH WATER DO YOU NEED A DAY?

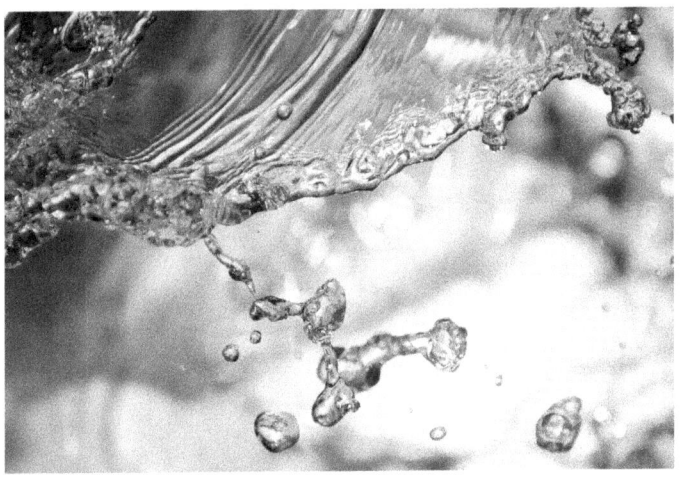

https://pixabay.com/en/splashing-splash-aqua-water-rain-165192/

How much water should you drink each day? It's a simple question with no easy answers. Our body is about 75% water, give or take. Water is an important structural component of skin cartilage, tissues and organs. For human beings, every part of the body is dependent on water.

However, we're constantly losing water from our bodies, primarily via urine and sweat.

Our body comprises about 75% water: the brain has 85%, blood is 90%, muscles are 75%, kidney is 82% and bones are 22% water. The functions of our glands and organs will eventually deteriorate if they are not nourished with good, clean water.

"Drink eight 8-ounce glasses of water a day." Its popular because it's easy to remember. Just keep in mind that the rule should be reframed as: "Drink eight 8-ounce glasses of fluid a day," because all fluids count toward the daily total.

IMPROVE HEALTH BY THROWING HATRED

Keeping on worried about the past and having anxiety about the future, the present naturally is affected. The best policy should be, to forget the past and have no anxiety about the future for which no one has control; the present has to be enjoyed at its best. The hatred towards self and others will be the most dangerous for the health, and it leads to not only unpleasantness but also develops hypertension and that will be the cause for setback of health. Imagine a situation that the vegetables in the house are unused for days together; naturally it rots and starts smelling you can tolerate for a while but not for long and it compels you to throw it away and have nice atmosphere. Similarly the hatred within us will cause such damage and it is better we throw as quickly as possible and be positive.

It is the time for all of us to throw away any hatred for anyone from your heart so that you will not carry sins for a lifetime. Forgiving others is the best attitude to take!

IDEAL MENU AND TIMINGS

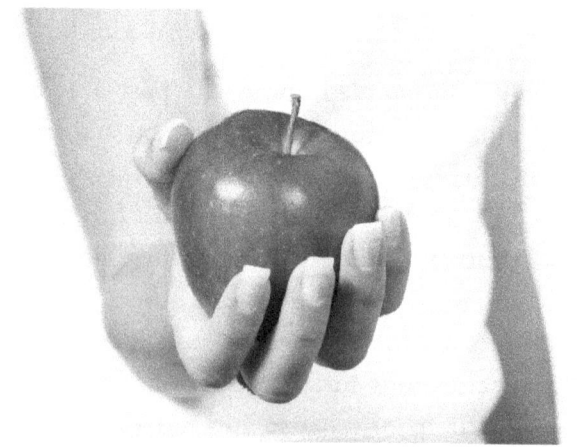

https://pixabay.com/en/apple-diet-female-food-fresh-2391/

- Drink 2 glasses of normal water on waking up early in the morning.
- Take a glass of juice preferably carrot or apple, before/after brisk walk around 7.00 am (During summer at 6.00 am).
- You may also take a cup of hot skimmed milk after vigorous yogic exercises, if it suits.
- Take good lunch (light but nutritious) as you need enough energy for working whole day. Lunch should be taken at 12:00 pm.

- A proper lunch should consists of -

Salad – To be consumed first
Cooked vegetables of 2 or 3 cups,
Medium sized chapatti- 2 or 3 or 2 bowls of Rice
Yoghurt(Dahi) 1 cup.
Steamed vegetables or Dal - ½ or 1 cup)

Note: Chapatti/Bread and rich should not be consumed together.

Around 2.00 pm

2 apples or 2 bananas or 2 pears or some papaya or any other fruit, but one variety only.

Supper (Around 7.00 pm)

Out of total 1600 calories consumed during the whole day, evening meal should not contain more than 350 calories.

As per your taste, and choice but it should be light,

e.g 1 or 2 cooked vegetables with 1 chapatti and 1 cup of yoghurt

1 cup of soup, 1 fruit and raw vegetables or

2 cups of skimmed milk with 1 or 2 bananas or apples or toast or bread slices.

Soups, fruits, salad/vegetables should be taken before meals and never before 2-3 hours.

Note: If you have to go out for dinner, take just a cup of skimmed milk or soup or eat some roasted grams or some fruits/vegetables at around 6.00pm before going. If you take a late evening dinner, drink a glass of lemon juice (juice of 1 lemon is one glass of warm water) the following morning (empty stomach)

HERBS AND SPICES

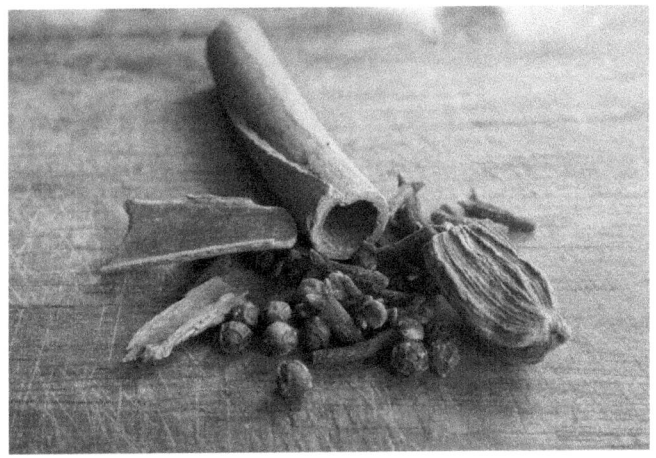

https://pixabay.com/en/spices-india-exotic-food-cinnamon-166903/

You may use asafoetida (hing), cloves, coriander, garlic, ginger, saunf, turmeric, cumin (jeera) cardamom, ajwain, pepper, kali rai and mint (pundina)

Fresh vegetables by way of green salad could be consumed plenty and less of cooked food. Imagine that the animals eat raw food and they are health and active.

Dry fruits are good substitute for the cooked food, practice be made to live on dry fruits at least for few days in a month.

Caution: Bed tea/ coffee is very harmful. Avoid tea / coffee / aerated / cold drinks, fried items always.

YOGA IS DIVINE

Yoga poses have been evolved and developed over centuries of research and experience. They have been found to be extremely effective in:

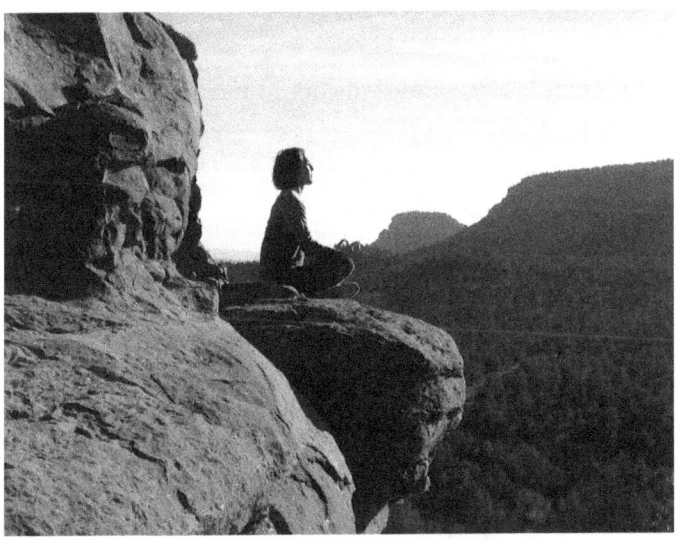

https://pixabay.com/en/peaceful-yoga-meditation-lifestyle-442070/

- Increasing flexibility of the body and freeing all the energy blocks. Thus leads to a healthier body.
- Helping to lose excess flab and weight - another cause of ill health.

- Massaging the internal organs of the body
- Helping to treat several health disorders - from common ones such as backaches and arthritis to 'seemingly' unrelated disorders such as stammering.

It is recommended to include some form of yoga positions and preferably a yoga routine in your life.

Meditation, Pranayama (Breathing), Relaxation and Cleansing

A complete yoga session should include these aspects which results in HUGE benefits in terms of:

- Correcting metabolic disorders.
- Overcoming stress and mind behaviors that seem beyond your control.
- Changing firmly entrenched attitudes or personality disorders.

COMMON SYMPTOMS OF HEART ATTACK...

A serious note about heart attacks - You should know that not every heart attack symptom is going to be the left arm hurting. Be aware of intense pain in the jaw line. You may never have the first chest pain during the course of a heart attack. Nausea and intense sweating are also common symptoms. 60% of people who have a heart attack while they are asleep do not wake up. Pain in the jaw can wake you from a sound sleep. Let's be careful and be aware. The more we know the better chance we could survive. One can avoid Heart attack with regular Yoga & Pranayama.

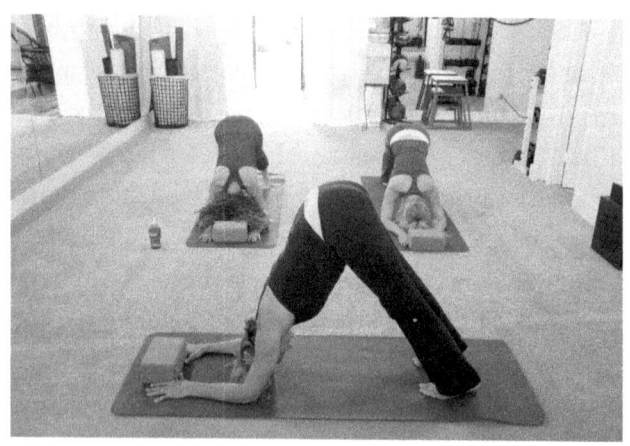

https://pixabay.com/en/yoga-workout-exercise-stretching-263673/

HEART ATTACH

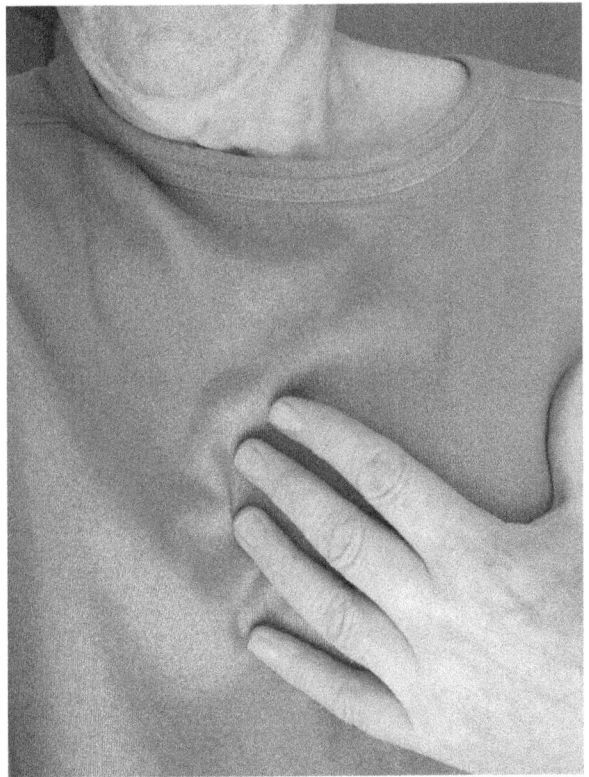

https://pixabay.com/en/body-upper-body-hand-t-shirt-keep-116585/

Heart Attacks And Drinking Warm Water

Not only about the warm water after your meal, but about Heart Attacks. The Chinese and Japanese drink hot tea with their meals, not cold water, maybe it is time we adopt their drinking habit while eating.

For those who like to drink cold water, this article is applicable to you. It is nice to have a cup of cold drink after a meal. However, the cold water will solidify the oily stuff that you have just consumed. It will slow down the digestion. Once this 'sludge' reacts with the acid, it will break down and be absorbed by the intestine faster than the solid food. It will line the intestine. Very soon, this will turn into fats and lead to cancer. It is best to drink hot soup or warm water after a meal.

Hardening or blockage of arteries leads to heart attack

Intake of foods containing Vitamin B6, Vitamin E and Magnesium be increased.

Contented and happy people can resist the onset of heart attack and other grave diseases.

Rich factors are:

Blood pressure, Diabetes, Cigarette smoking, Blood cholesterol, Overweight, Nil exercise and Sedentary habits.

Symptoms of Heart attack are:

Chest pain, Difficulty in breathing, Profuse perspiration, Nausea, Vomitting and Mental tension, Feeling very weak.

Disorders:

Blood circulation, Digestive, Respiratory.

It takes two to three months for the heart to heal.

During your life time, your heart will beat almost 3 billion times and pumps enough blood to fill 100 swimming pools.

HOW TO HANDLE STRESS

One cannot avoid stress. Doing regular exercise and sufficient sleep will help body's resistance to stress. By relaxing, resting, taking a walk, meditating and many other things to suit the moods, the stress could be reduced. Stress is nothing but mental and physical illness. If stress is not handled properly, it can lead to many complications. Prolonged stress will contribute to serious health problems like Blood Pressure, Diabetic, Stomach Ulcers, etc. One should try to eliminate or diminish the stress by sharing the problems with a friend, relative or well wisher, which would help release stress.

Yoga helps you copy with this stress so that you do not need to depend on smoking or eating unhealthy food. It also helps you find contentment from within. Smoking should be completely stopped as it constricts the arteries.

For daily practice:

- Keep yourself relaxed and free from anxiety, nervousness, tension and restlessness.

- Meditation has been scientifically proven to be beneficial for hypertensive people.
- Ujjavi Pranayam can be done while lying for about 3-4 minutes, if the blood pressure rises very high.
- Nadi Shodak Pranayam can be done 10 times.
- Yoga contains elements that address problems at every level.
- Asanas that relax and tone our muscles and massage our internal organs.
- Pranayama slows our breathing and regulates the flow of prana relaxation and meditation that act to calm our mind and equanimity.
- Daily practice of yoga can restore our natural balance and harmony – physical, mental and spiritual.

GOLDEN RULES FOR GOOD LIFE

The posture of Sitting, standing and sleeping should be proper.

Do Regular exercises for the whole body especially for back exercise.

Take breaks periodically i.e. do not sit or stand for longer duration.

Use proper chair with lumbar support.

Do not use high heel shoes.

Drink plenty of water.

Walk as much as possible.

Practice yoga & pranayama regularly.

Do not eat beyond your limits& needs.

PHYSICAL FITNESS

Physical fitness and good health are complimentary to each other. Physically fit people perform better, have more energy, look better, feel good, etc. Physical fitness increases the efficiency and capacity of the heart and lungs also help to maintain and control weight. They have greater resistance to disease and recover faster from illness. More than all happiness, alertness resist the effects of ageing and relaxation is in built in physical fitness.

HOW TO KEEP FIT

Health Tips

- One Apple /Day – No Doctor
- One Tulsi Leaf /Day – No Cancer
- One Lemon /Day – No Fat
- One cup Milk /Day – No Bone Problem
- 3 ltr Water /Day – No Diseases

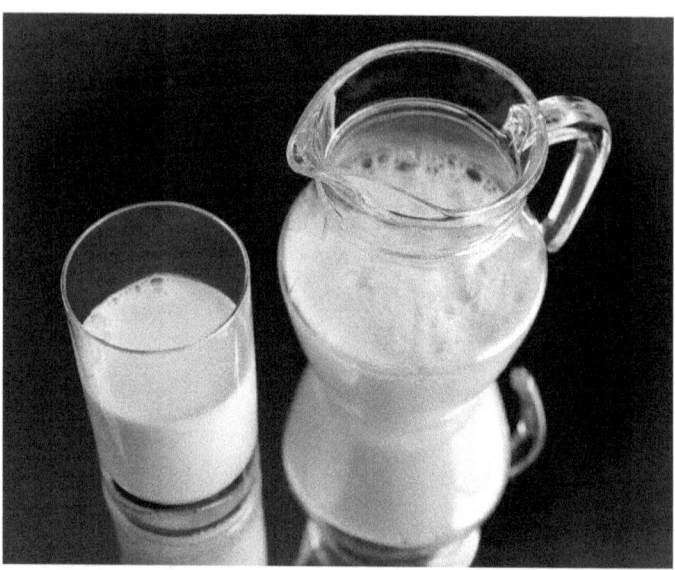

https://pixabay.com/en/milk-glass-frisch-healthy-drink-518067/

Walking, Jogging, Exercising, Jim, Hiking, Running such activities should be made as routine to have good physical fitness.

In order to have better physical fitness, one should be active and involve in any sport like, Tennis, Badminton, Cricket, Football, Basketball, Table Tennis, Golf, Snooker or any sport which not only keeps the body fit but there will be full relaxation for the mind.

Alternatively the activities such as Fishing, Dancing of any kind, Dusting, Mopping, Sweeping, Cleaning etc., could be attended.

If none of the above could be done at least the following activities be undertaken:

1. Kids' games. Join the grandkids for a game of hopscotch, tag or red rover.

2. Water polo. For those who like their swimming mixed with competitive fun.

3. Mowing. If your lawn is small enough to use an unpowered push mower, the workout is even better.

4. Raking. For twice the exercise, rake the leaves; jump into the pile and then rake them again.

5. Rock/shell collecting. One way to give a purpose to long walks.

6. Rowing. It's great because you can always follow exercise with a few hours of fishing.

7. Softball. Try the slow-pitch version for the thrill of baseball without the 90-mph pitches.

42 CA. Dr. Vishnu Bharath Alampalli

8. Stair climbing. Beats waiting for that slow elevator again.

9. Stationary cycling. As you pedal in place, you can even read a book or watch some TV.

10. Swimming. With the water bearing your weight, swimming is easy on the bones and joints.

11. Table tennis. It's a lot less running than full-size tennis but still good exercise.

12. Walking. The king of all fitness activities: cheap, easy and convenient. And it works, too.

13. Water aerobics. Sign up for a class at your local pool. You'll be glad you did.

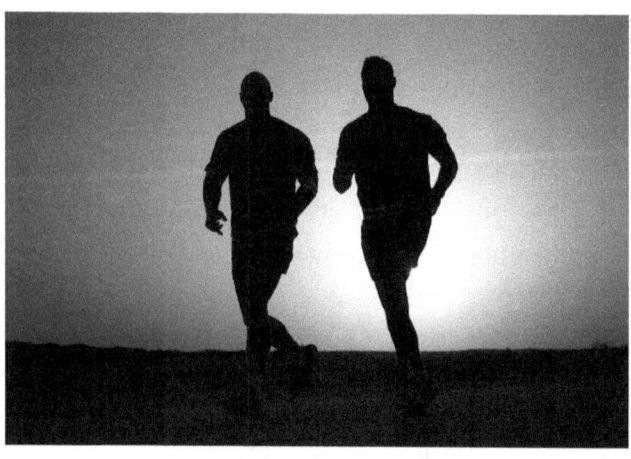

https://pixabay.com/en/runners-silhouettes-athletes-635906/

HOW TO KEEP FIT:

Exercise

1. An act of employing or putting into play; use: the free exercise of intellect; the exercise of an option.
2. Activity that requires physical or mental exertion, especially when performed to develop or maintain fitness: took an hour of vigorous daily exercise at a gym.

Tips for exercising

Always wear appropriate gear, such as the appropriate shoes for each sport.

- Warm up before exercising. This can be a moderate activity such as walking at your normal pace while emphasizing arm movements.
- Exercise at least 30 minutes a day. You can split this into periods of 10 to 15 minutes.
- Make sure you drink enough water. You can be dehydrated without feeling thirsty.
- Never increase your program more than 10 percent a week. This applies to the distance you walk or the amount of weight you lift, for instance.
- Consider varying your routine. Mixing tennis and weight lifting, for example, offers different workouts and keeps exercise interesting.

- When using exercise equipment, read instructions carefully and, if needed, ask a qualified person for help. Make sure equipment is in good working order.
- Stop exercising if you experience severe pain or swelling. Persistent discomfort should always be evaluated.

Sport

1. Physical activity that is governed by a set of rules or customs and often engaged in competitively.
2. An activity involving physical exertion and skill that is governed by a set of rules or customs and often undertaken competitively.

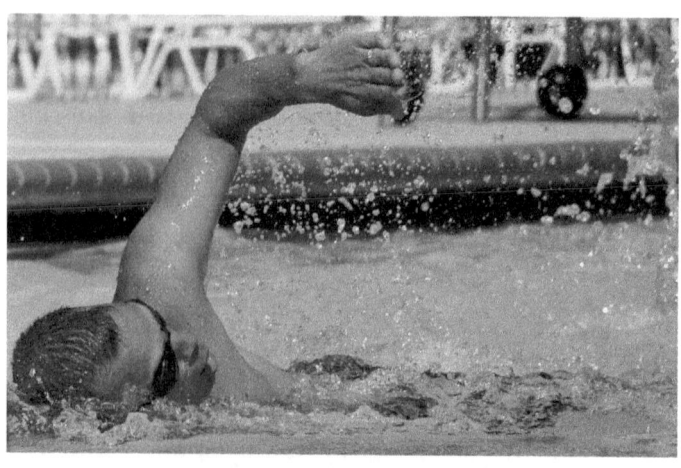

https://pixabay.com/en/
swimmer-pool-water-swimming-stroke-802891/

Swimming

Swimming is the act of moving through water by using the arms and legs. The whole body gets exercise and more than all the body floats in coolant. Swimming is one of the best exercise for keeping physically fit. Swimming improves heart actions, aids blood circulation and also helps to develop firm muscles. Different types of swimming include freehand, backstroke, butterfly, breaststroke and sidestroke.

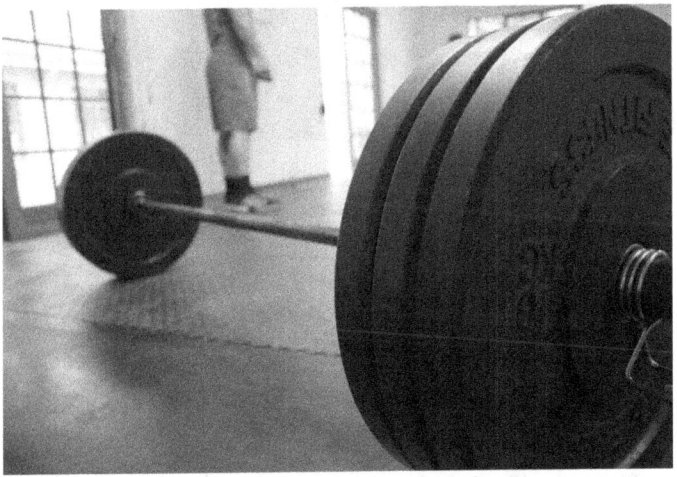

https://pixabay.com/en/gym-barbell-training-exercise-592899/

Gymming

Physical exercises designed to develop and display strength, balance, and agility, especially those performed on or with specialized apparatus.

b. Practice or training in exercises that develop physical strength and agility or mental capacity

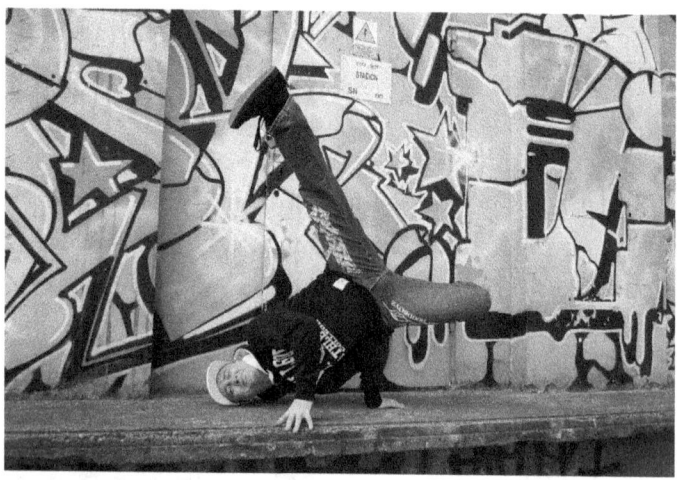

https://pixabay.com/en/dance-body-breakdance-559885/

Dancing

To move with measured steps, or to a musical accompaniment; to go through, either alone or in company with others, with a regulated succession of movements, (commonly) to the sound of music; to trip or leap rhythmically. To move nimbly or merrily; to express pleasure by motion; to caper; to frisk; to skip about.

The leaping, tripping, or measured stepping of one who dances; an amusement, in which the movements of the persons are regulated by art, in figures and in accord with music.

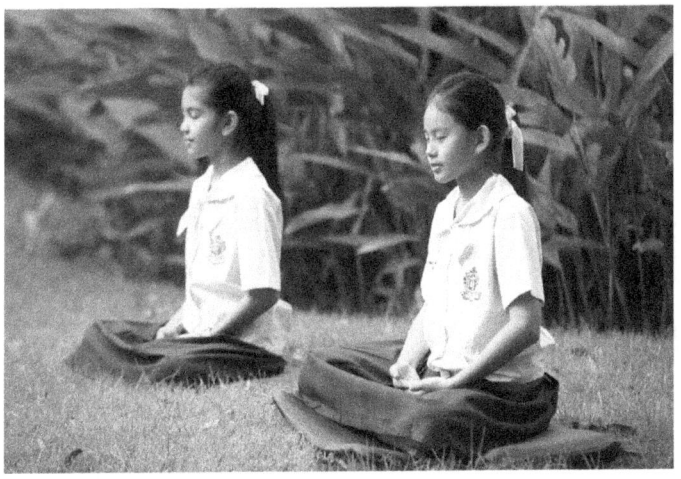

https://pixabay.com/en/girls-buddhism-meditation-481261/

Meditation

Meditation means awareness. Whatever you do with awareness is meditation.

Meditation is conscious sleep and Sleep is un conscious meditation.

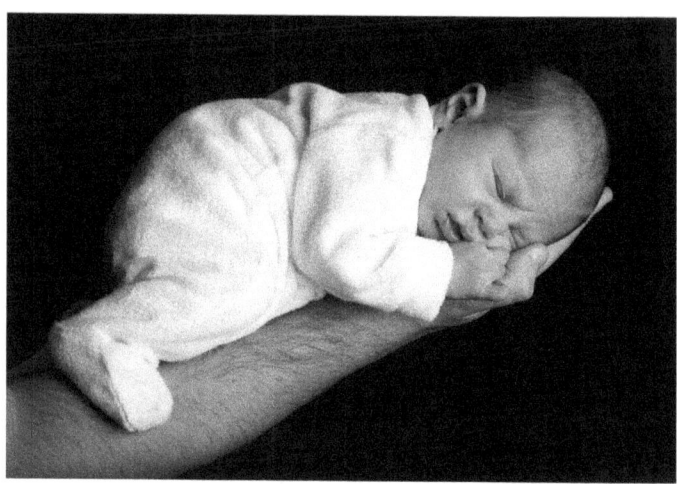

https://pixabay.com/en/baby-care-child-cute-hand-face-20339/

Rest & Sleep

To overcome fatigue and restore energy to the body, one needs rest and sleep. Rest / sleep of 6-8 hours per day is adequate.

WHY IT IS GOOD TO SMILE

SMILE/ LAUGHTER WILL REMOVE STRESS, MAKE BEST USE OF IT:

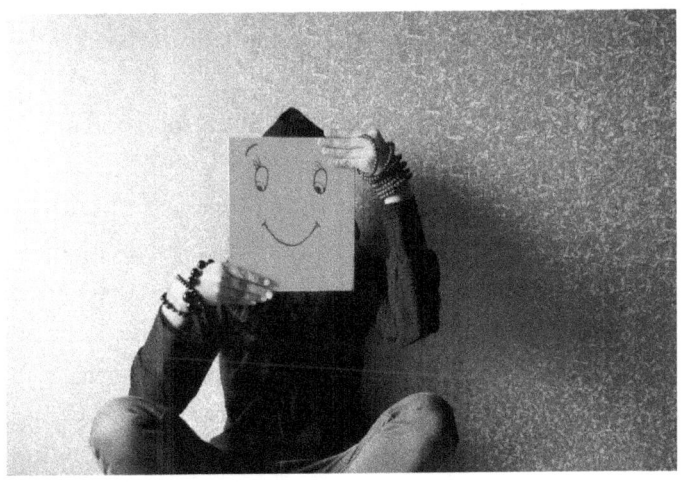

https://pixabay.com/en/man-happy-face-smiley-mask-390342/

"Even if there is nothing to laugh about, laugh on credit."

Even a child can understand SMILE. What you cannot achieve by using tons of money, you could achieve in a simple smile, one should cultivate the habit of smiling on every situation and this will remove the stress. There are 19 types of smile and it could be different categories such as Polite, Social, casual, formal, normal and natural. Smile use more muscles on both sides of the face. Smile costs nothing but creates much. Be happy and make others happy should be your motto, putting on a happy face is absolutely good for you, and those around you. For thousands of years; it has been acknowledged that "Laughter is the best Medicine". It is proved in scientific research that it has many beneficial effects of humor on health. Laughter can come in handy, whether it's for dealing with an illness, the pressures of daily living, stress, coping at work even, laughter can dramatically change the quality and outlook of our lives.

A smile/laugh, whatever you call it is too good and it enhance your mood, health, fitness etc.,

Laughter helps in many ways to improve the health by reducing the level of stress hormones. Laughter enhances number of antibody –producing cells, enhance good hormones. Laughter is good for not only brain but also for Heart and it relaxes the body to be more active and at tentative. Laughter removes the anger stress, guilt and negative emotions and make you positive frame of mind and make you cheerful. Laughing self and others around will make things better and as for as possible the laughter should be natural and one can laugh unnatural but it will not have same effect as natural laughter. Imagine, no other living creature can express feelings better than humans and humans are bestowed to express, laugh, communicate and what not. It is better we realize the advantage of laughter and start to have laughing as regular and as more frequent at possible.

WHY ARE YOU KEEPING QUITE, LAUGH & SMILE TO YOUR HEART'S CONTENT?

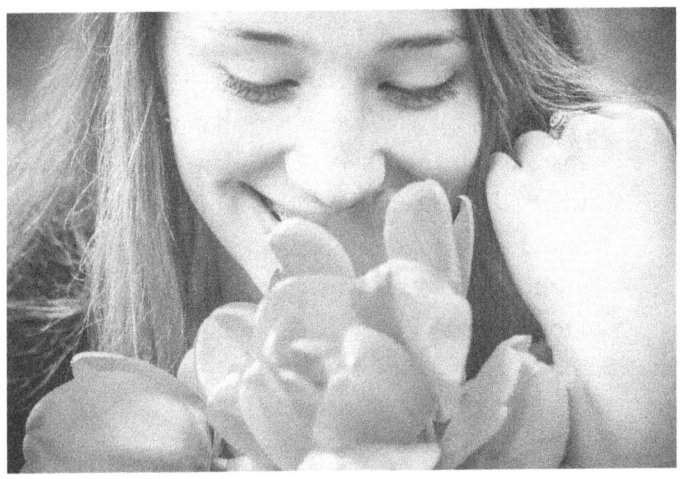

https://pixabay.com/en/girl-spring-smile-photographer-777468/

HOW TO USE LAUGHTER:

- Laugh with friends: Going to a movie or comedy club with friends is a great way to get more laughter in your life. Having friends over for a party or game night is also a great setup for laughter and other good feelings.
- Find humor in your life: Instead of complaining about life's frustrations, try to laugh about them.
- TV and movies: When you feel like laugh, don't control when you are seeing TV program or cinema in the theater and viewing in the video. Choose such programs that it makes you laugh.

- "Fake it, till you make it!": Just as studies show the positive effects of smiling occur whether the smile is fake or real, faked laughter also provides the benefits mentioned above. So smile more, and fake laughter; you'll still achieve positive effects.
- Laughing invokes feelings of happiness and joy. Instead of being all gloomy and frustrated because there is no perceived solution, laughing lifts us up out of our pool of problems and plops us on solid ground where we can gain some new insights. Don't forget to LOL (laugh out loud) frequently!

The Benefits of Smiling

- Here are the many social, physical and mental benefits that something as simple as a smile can do! A smile can...
- Make you look younger.
- Fill you up with positivity and power.
- Show your understanding side.
- Say that you can be polite in the hardest of times.
- Help you live longer.
- Make you appreciate the little things in life.
- Make you look at the brighter side of a bad situation.
- Be contagious to all those around you.
- Start your day pleasantly.
- Make others understand you are in a good mood.
- Promote positivity in a work environment.
- Relax your face muscles.

- Make others put a smile on their face.
- Tell people that they are going to be okay.
- Makes you look a lot prettier or more handsome.
- Reduce all of that stress you might accumulate.
- Help your immune system work a lot better.
- Lower your blood pressure.
- Give you a child like innocence.
- Release serotonin, natural pain killers and endorphins thus making it a happy drug.

A smile has more wonderful benefits that you could ever think about.

I know that after you've read this, you are smiling now so don't let anything stop it because a smile is like eating 2000 bars of chocolate! So happy smiling!

We could all do with a bit of cheering up every now and then, so with research suggesting that all we need to do is smile, we look at how a simple facial expression could help lighten your mood.

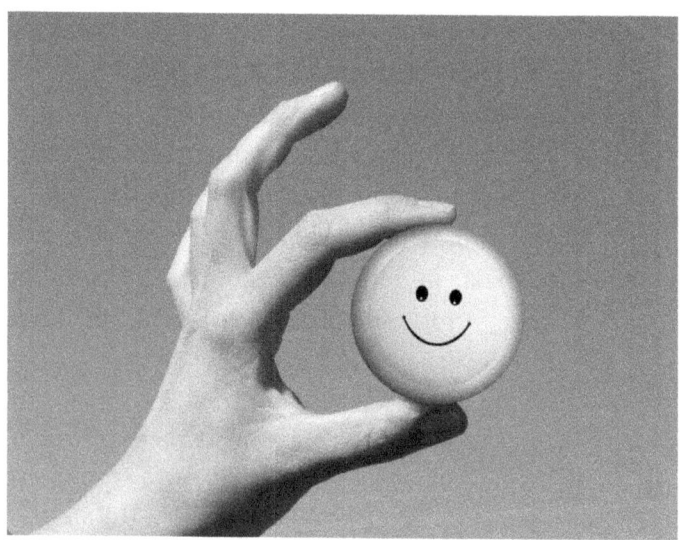

https://pixabay.com/en/smiley-emoticon-hand-finger-keep-237145/

Why it's good to smile

Smiling, laughing, and positive thinking have been shown to have a huge number of health benefits to both mind and body.

Stress has been linked to a number of health problems, including heart disease, Type 2 diabetes, high blood pressure and obesity.

A good laugh can be beneficial to the lungs, boost immunity, and could even burn off calories.

Smiley, happy people are thought to have more friends and be more successful, by appearing more confident and approachable.

When you laugh, your body releases endorphins. They are also a natural pain and stress reliever.

Laughing reduces levels of cortisol, the stress hormone, and gives us a quick burst of energy.

OIL BATH & IT'S ADVANTAGES

It is age old and proven beyond doubt, that the Oil bath and massage relax the body and it is better to have often as frequent as possible. Massaging could be from different type of oil may be Ginger, Caster, sesame, coconut or mixed oil and instantly it removes the stress and helps for better physical fitness. Regular massage of body makes the body and skin smooth and enhances the moisture in the body. Especially people living in hot climatic conditions have to go for massaging as frequent as possible.

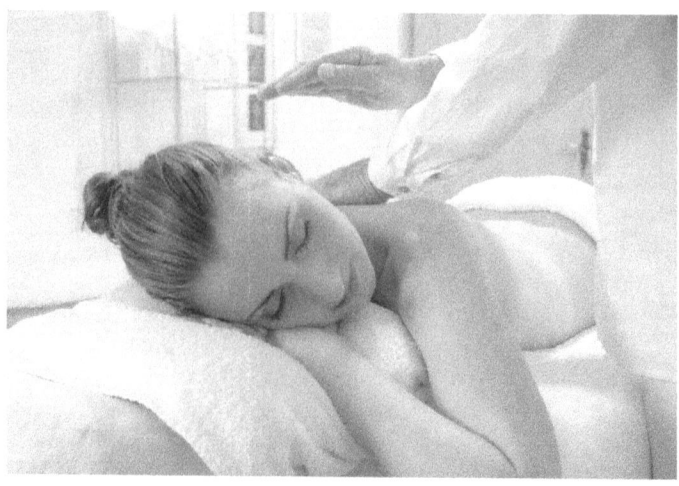

https://pixabay.com/en/wellness-massage-relax-relaxing-285587/

EATING A FRUIT

FRUITS SHOULD BE EATEN ON EMPTY STOMACH i.e BEFORE LUNCH/DINNER.

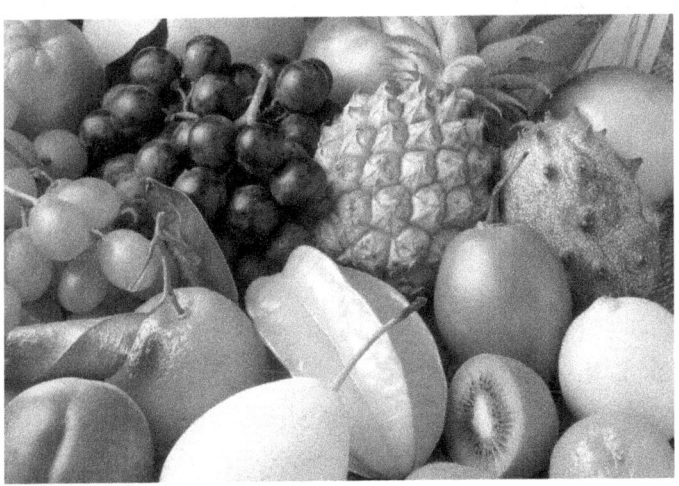

https://pixabay.com/en/fruits-sweet-fruit-exotic-82524/

Most of us eat fruits after a heavy meal and satisfied that after all the fruits can be digested fast and it does not matter if you take it even after the heavy meal is not at all correct and in fact you have to eat fruit on empty stomach. There is logic behind this and could be proved scientifically. THEREFORE IT MEANS NOT EATING FRUITS AFTER YOUR MEALS! FRUITS

SHOULD BE EATEN ON AN EMPTY STOMACH, i.e. before meal.

If you eat fruit like that, it will play a major role to detoxify your system, supplying you with a great deal of energy for weight loss and other life activities. It is known fact that fruits get digested quickly and the solid food we take time to digest. Just take example that the heavy lunch is taken and as desert the fruits are taken after the food. The solid food taken is stored for digestion and the fruits taken will land up on the solid food which is yet to be digested and by the time it takes for digestion of solid food, the fruits get rot inside the stomach and naturally the solid food also get rot and it has its own effect.

Now take it other way, by taking the fruits in the beginning i.e before the solid food, it allows for easy digestion and also the stomach is filled and the solid food taken will be less to that extent and the solid food will takes its natural time to digest without getting rot inside the stomach.

Most unfortunately, our ancestors may be they did not realize and it is age old practice to take fruits at the end. It is even more worse to take ice cream after the solid food and fruits, as it freezes out the entire block and get more time to digest, and results in stomach upset. It is idle to take fruits and ice cream in the beginning and the solid food latter and at the end to take hot soup which eases out the food for quick digestion. The problems like graying hair, balding, nervous outburst, and dark circles under the eyes all these will NOT happen if you take fruits on an empty stomach.

There is belief that some fruits, like orange and lemon are acidic, because all fruits become alkaline in our body. If it is followed on regular basis the intake as indicated above one will see their face is glowing, enhances the beauty, longevity, health, energy, happiness and normal weight.

It is always better to eat fruits in its physical form by nicely cleaning and cutting it and not by making into juice. Another important thing is to eat fresh fruits and definitely not processed, cooked etc., as it loses nutrients. Of course it is better to drink the fresh fruit juice than battled juice or caned juice as the processed juice is not fresh and it loses the vital vitamins. Even drinking the fresh fruit juice, it would be slowly consumed and the juice be mixed with saliva which enables to cleanse the body. Just to be on fruits/fruit juice once in a while, pulls you down the weight and the face becomes elegant and radiant you look.

Each type of fruit has its own specialties and best among are Orange, Apple, Strabery, Kiwi, watermelon, Guava, Papaya

Drinking Cold water after a meal, leads to Cancer! Can u believe this? For those who like to drink cold water, this article is applicable to you. It is nice to have a cup of cold drink after a meal. However, the cold water will solidify the oily stuff that you have just consumed. It will slow down the digestion. Once this 'sludge' reacts with the acid, it will break down and be absorbed by the intestine faster than the solid food. It will line the intestine. Very soon, this will turn into fats and lead to cancer. It is best to drink hot soup or warm water after a meal.

BANANA IS SANJEEVANI (TOO GOOD)

Bananas is too good and it has lot of Glucose with fiber and natural sugar. A banana gives instantly, sustained and substantial boost of energy. Banana is popular all round the world and all athletes are encouraged to have banana as it gives sufficient energy. It can also help overcome or prevent a substantial number of illnesses and conditions, making it a must to add to our daily diet. Banana has high in iron, and it can stimulate the production of hemoglobin in the blood and so helps in cases of anemia. People who had gone for depression are fed with banana and lot of improvement was found as it has lot of protein to improve your mood and generally make you feel happier.

Banana is unique tropical fruit is extremely high in potassium yet low in salt, making it the perfect to beat blood pressure.

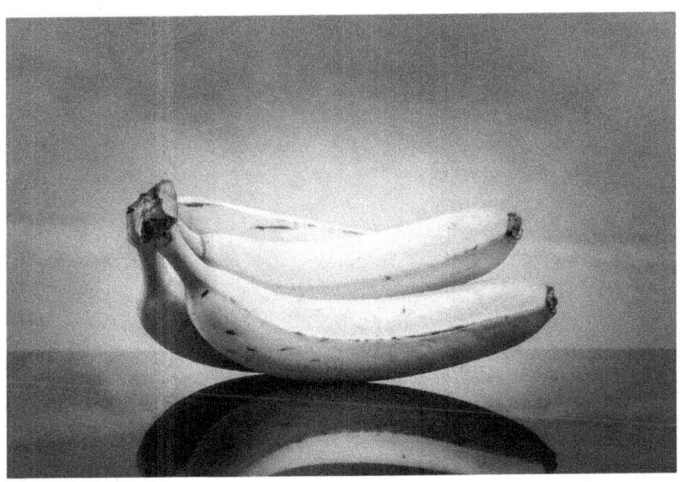

https://pixabay.com/en/banana-yellow-close-up-ripe-316649/

KILL THE ILL WITH OUT A PILL - HERBAL REMEDIES

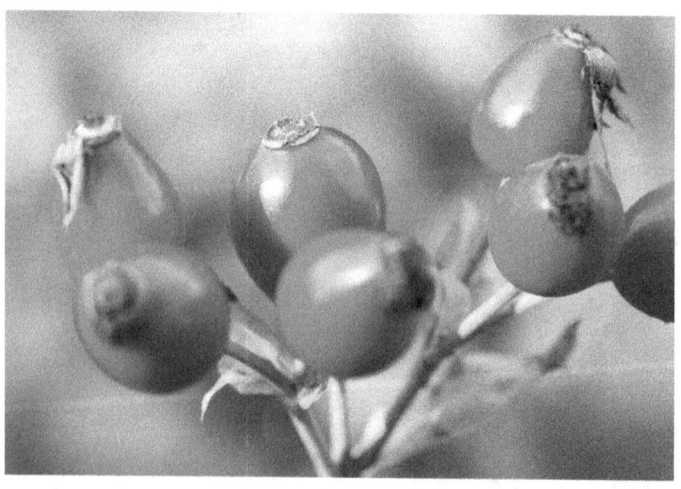

https://pixabay.com/en/rose-hip-canina-fruit-red-493784/

Health is so very important and most of us knowing or unknowingly Neglect, till something drastic health upset happens. The Creator Almighty gave precious life to humans, animals, birds and other living creatures and he was so great to give food to all from ant to elephant and all of them live peacefully and more importantly healthy, take for example the animals and birds eat raw food and live very actively without shelter, clothing etc., they don't have hospitals or Doctors to treat them and on contrary humans, being very brainy, have changed the food habits from time to time, did experiments and found different type of food by spoiling the naturality. By boiling, roosting, smashing, frying, mixing etc., and this had led to detrition of health.

OREGANO helps soothe stomach muscles.

MINT can ease hiccups.

GINGER is anti-nausea remedy.

FENUGREEK helps flush out harmful toxins.

FENNEL can reduce bad breath and body odor.

SAGE is antiseptic & antibiotic.

THYME relaxes respiratory muscles.

TURMERIC is anti-cancer.

BASIL can relieve gas and soothe stomach upsets.

BLACK PEPPER helps relieve indigestion.

CAYENNE can stop a heart attack.

CINNAMON helps lower blood pressure.

DILL will treat heartburn, colic and gas.

ROSEMARY is antioxidant.

CHERRIES help calm nervous system.

GRAPES relax blood vessels.

PEACHES have Potassium & Iron.

APPLES help resistance against infections.

WATERMELON help control heart rate.

ORANGES help maintain skin & vision.

STRAWBERRIES fight against cancer and aging.

BANANAS gives lot of energy.

PINAPPLE help fight arthritis.

BLUEBERRIES protect Heart.

KIWIES increase bone mass.

MANGOS protect cancer.

HEALTHY DRINKS FOR TOTAL WELLNESS

TO BOOST ENERGY & CLEAN SYSTEM: CARROT+GINGER+AOOLE JUICE.

TO PREVENT CANCER & REDUCE CHOLESTEROL: APPLE+CUCUMBER+CELERY JUICE.

TO IMPROVE SKIL COMPLEXION & BAD BRETH: TOMATO+CARROT+ APPLE JUICE.

TO REDUCE INTERNAL BODY HEAT: BITTER GUARD+APPLE+MILK.

TO REDUCE BODY HEAT & SKIN TEXTURE: ORANGE+GINGER+CUCUMBER.

TO DISPEL EXCESS SALT & CLEAN BLADDER/KIDNEY: PINEAPPLE+APPLE+WATERMELON.

TO IMPROVE SKIN COMPLEXION: APPLE+CUCUMBER+KIWI FRUIT JUICE.

TO REGULATE SUGAR CONTENT: PEAR & BANANA.

TO REDUCE BLOOD PLEASSURE: CARROT+APPLE+PEAR+MANGO JUICE.

TO STRENTHEN BODY IMMUNITY:
HONEYDEW+GRAPS+WATERMELON+MILK.

TO IMPROVE METABOLISM:
PAPAYA+PINEAPPLE+MILK.

TO PREVENT CONSTIPATION:
BANANA+PINEAPPLE+MILK.

All RED FRUITS protect against HEART DISEASE,

Prevent BLOOD CLOTS & improve BLOOD
CIRCULATION.

RED FRUITS have rich Antioxidants which not
only gives red color to body and also protect against
CANCER DISEASES.

HOW TO CONTROL THE FOOD INTAKE

90% OF Energy is derived from only 10% of food eaten, then why over eat? Do not eat when under emotional stress or when extremely fatigue. Do not swallow until the food have been thoroughly masticated, as stomach do not have teeth and the food you take is the medicine for providing the required energy. There are many physiological and Psychological mechanisms which are thought to contribute to the control of our food intake. Most of which are thought to be co-ordinated through the integration of various complex systems involving parts of the brain, stomach, liver, hormones and other chemicals within the blood. More research is needed into these complex processes to enable us to fully understand the detailed workings behind them. The following list shows some of the simpler control mechanisms that we do understand, some are within our control but others are determined by our genetics.

PHYSICAL ACTIVITY

NUTRITION FOR ENERGY

In order to <u>lose weight</u> good nutrition is important it helps optimize the body's energy system to work efficiently so exercise can be more effective. When people try to lose weight many reduce their <u>food intake</u> dramatically, eventually the nutritional status becomes low. As the body <u>burns fat</u> or <u>carbohydrates</u> the cells require essential nutrients to complete the chemical process. An imbalance in the nutritional state very often affects energy levels, the result is we may feel low and drained of energy!

Obviously the muscles don't become paralyzed from deficiencies in certain vitamins or minerals but an imbalance can affect us in different ways. Have you ever had that feeling where you want to get up and <u>exercise to lose weight</u> but your body just don't seem to want to know, you begin to <u>workout</u> and within five minutes you feel drained or even faint!

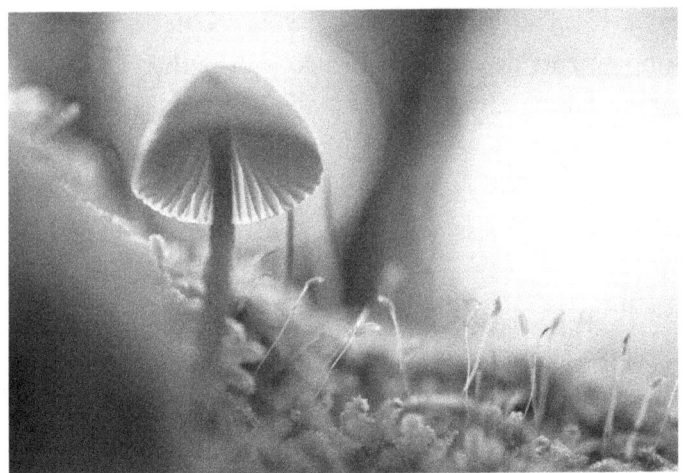

https://pixabay.com/en/nature-mushroom-closeup-macro-hat-768563/

Nutritional Facts

Many of the <u>B vitamins</u> are required for the process of <u>energy metabolism</u>. If a reduced calorie diet does not provide enough B vitamins the <u>metabolism of fats</u> and carbohydrates may be affected and result in a feeling of lethargy.

<u>Vitamin C</u> not only helps fight resistance to infections it also helps repair and maintain muscle tissue and blood vessels. Stronger lean body tissue is essential in order to <u>exercise</u> long enough to burn sufficient calories for <u>permanent weight loss</u>.

Its not necessary to buy tons of vitamin and mineral pills just to ensure you obtain all essential nutrients. Taking one multi-vitamin pill each day should be plenty to help keep up energy levels so you can exercise effectively, however if you decide to take any supplements do remember to consult with your doctor before taking any.

Sufficient quality protein is also necessary to limit loss of lean body tissue when losing weight. The less lean tissue loss the less a reduction in the basal metabolic rate.

Proper nutrition means providing all the components - protein, carbohydrate, essential fatty acids, vitamins, minerals and electrolytes. The body can last for a long time on a calorie reduced diet but requires a regular supply of essential nutrients to help the body use stored energy - body fat!

DIET

The right food maintains health while the wrong food produces disease. Eat only when you are hungry, never over eat should be the principal. Diet is the food and drink that a person takes regularly. Diet varies according to age, weight, condition of health, climate and activity. A balanced diet contains proteins to build tissues, fat and carbohydrates to provide energy and heat. Minerals and vitamins are needed for growth and to regulate body functions.

Food is one of our most basic needs. Food gives us the energy for everything such as walking, talking, working, playing, reading, thinking and breathing. Food also provides energy to nerves, muscles, heart and glands. The food mainly comes out of plants such as grains, fruits and vegetables. Food out of plants are healthy barring very few. Food from animals, which include meat, eggs and dairy products. The cost of food from animals are much more than the cost of food from the plants that also difficult to digest and rich in cholesterol content. However, the flesh of fish is proven to be a healthy food. The kind of food that people eat, vary from one country to another and sometimes even within the country. The food vary due to geographical reasons i.e. location, climate, physical features, etc. It also vary due to economic reasons, religious reasons, customs, etc.

Fresh food to consume is always good, tasty and healthy. The frozen food no doubt prevents the growth of microorganisms but considered not very healthy as compared to fresh food.

Control of our food intake is the basis behind successful weight loss.

CLEAN YOUR KIDNEYS

Years pass by and our kidneys are filtering the blood by removing salt, poison and any unwanted entering our body. With time, the salt accumulates and this needs to undergo cleaning treatments.

It is very easy, first take a bunch of parsley (KOTHIMBIR, HARA DHANIYA) and wash it clean then cut it in small pieces and put it in a pot and pour clean water and boil it for ten minutes and let it cool down and then filter it and pour in a clean bottle and keep it inside refrigerator to cool. Drink one glass daily and you will notice all salt and other accumulated poison coming out of your kidney by urination. Also you will be able to notice the difference which you never felt before. Parsley is known as best cleaning treatment for kidneys and it is natural!

NATURAL THERAPY FOR HEART VAIN OPENING

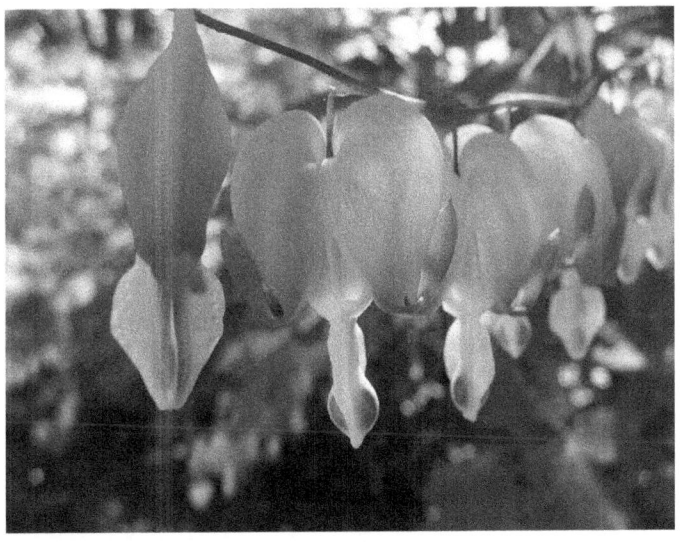

https://pixabay.com/en/bleeding-hearts-flowers-cluster-red-55120/

Heart Vein opening

On daily basis, every morning a glass of lemon juice with ginger, garlic and apple vinegar, heated up and mixed with pure honey, be consumed and it will help open the blockages in the blood flow.

Standard Blood Pressure: The standard blood pressure varies from person to person and most healthy sign is 120/70 to 140/90. The pressure varies depending upon the work, situation, circumstances etc., and to have same pressure in different conditions is welcome sign. The reading more than 140/90 indicates the need for medical intervention and guidance of a doctor.

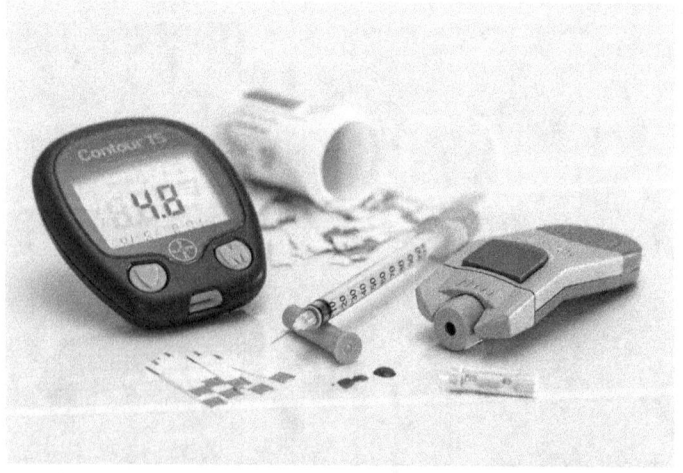

https://pixabay.com/en/diabetes-blood-sugar-diabetic-528678/

Range of Blood Sugar: Normally the sugar level in empty stomach, should be around 80 to 120 mg/dl. And after the food it should be between 120 to 160 mg/dl i.e after two hours of taking the food. The sugar level should come down to 100 to 140 mg/dl at the end of the day i.e bed time.

THE IMPORTANCE OF SLEEP!

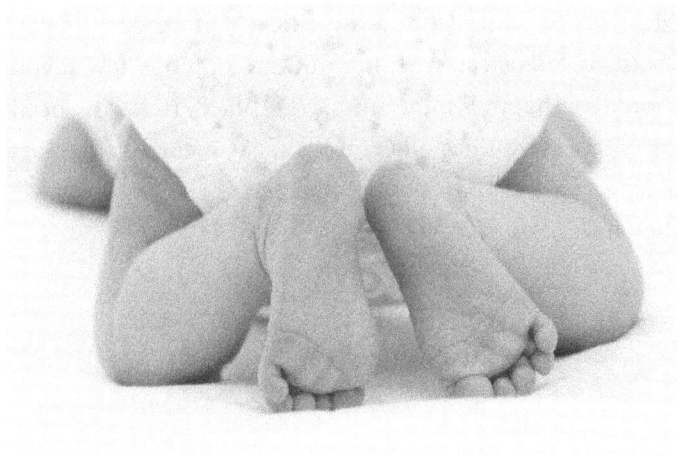

https://pixabay.com/en/baby-feet-cute-tiny-little-boy-218193/

Sleep is most essential in one's life, without food one can survive for few months but without sleep one will get restless and may collapse. The adult needs around 6/8 hours of sleep a night, but in practice actually people sleep more. Infants sleep about 14/16 hours a day, while teenagers need about 8 hours on average. Although some people claim that 4/5 hours of sound sleep is enough to keep fit. There is quite a bit of variation.

However, it is very difficult to pin down what is optimal for any particular person, as individual sleep needs can vary quite significantly. Some people are just naturally "long sleepers" or "short sleepers", and this does not constitute a <u>sleep disorder</u> of any sort, merely a genetic predilection, and daytime functioning in such individuals may be normal and healthy.

If you are drowsy during the day, even during boring periods, you haven't had enough sleep the previous night. Most people experience a dip in early afternoon. If you routinely fall asleep within 5 minutes of lying down, you should be happy. Sometimes you'll hear that you need less sleep as you get older. But that is incorrect. Seniors often sleep less than young adults and children because they have insomnia.

THE MAIN CAUSES OF LIVER DAMAGE

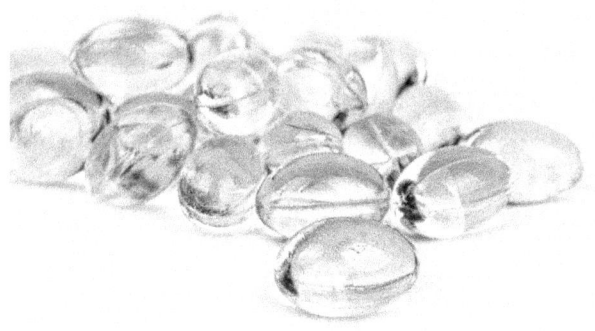

https://pixabay.com/en/pill-yellow-isolated-316601/

1. Sleeping too late and waking up too late are main cause.
2. Not urinating in the morning.
3. Too much eating.
4. Skipping breakfast.
5. Consuming too much medication.
6. Consuming too much preservatives, additives, food coloring, and artificial sweetener.
7. Consuming unhealthy cooking oil. As much as possible reduce cooking oil use when frying,

which includes even the best cooking oils like olive oil. Do not consume fried foods when you are tired, except if the body is very fit.

8. Consuming raw (overly done) foods also add to the burden of liver.

Veggies should be eaten raw or cooked 3-5 parts. Fried veggies should be finished in one sitting, do not store.

We should prevent this without necessarily spending more. We just have to adopt a good daily lifestyle and eating habits. Maintaining good eating habits and time condition are very important for our bodies to absorb and get rid of unnecessary chemicals according to 'schedule.'

HEAR FROM HORSES MOUTH: A BUSINESS MAN

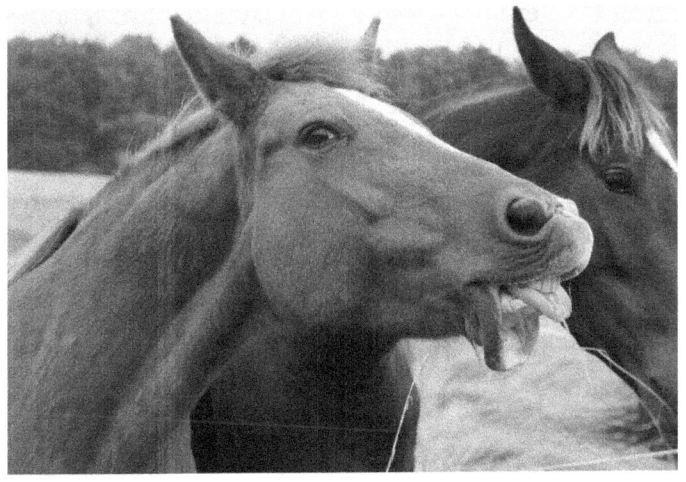

https://pixabay.com/en/horse-animal-pferdeportrait-659182/

I was born fat, I was tampered with rich food and I weighed 125 kgs by 40 years. My life style was such; I had no time for the proper exercise. My legs could not bear the weight, I started pain all over the body, and the day came that I was immobile. That is the day I took oath to reduce my weight and started my day at 5.30 a.m with one hour swimming and followed by 90 minutes Yoga. Instead of breakfast, I started Ragi Soup for the breakfast and took water in plenty to Kill my Diet. Latter I started only Fiber's food, vegetables and fruits. The Salt and Sugar was reduced to the barest minimum. It is my experience that with salt the food tastes better and you are tempted to eat more. Less of salt it does not taste good and you naturally reduce intake and that is sufficient to have energy for day to day work.

I also started following Naturopathy with regular exercise in evenings also and today after five months of rigorous follow up. I am proud for having reduced 25 kgs and feel very light and more energetic, always attentive and could work much better than before. Now it motivates me to reduce further 25 kgs to 75 kgs which will be standard for my height.

I always think that mind should control the body and not the body over the mind. I am more disciplined, smile comes out in my face as I do not have any pain of what so ever nature and daily, I check my weight and get enthused to see some grams are lost and that is for ever and never to add in my life.

Hear from Horses Mouth – A Software Engineer

It so happened that a very successful Software Engineer got heart attack and was rushed to Hospital, the Doctors made full investigation and found that there is blockage of 90% in the main artery and he was advised to go through the operation immediately. Naturally he was frightened and though of risk factor and also shared his life style he lead throughout and recommended to his fellow men/women that they should take care of their health utmost and not to neglect at any cost.

This was his life style......

1. He was only concentrating on the work and Slept in very odd timings, going to bed between 12:00 AM and 3:00 AM. Waking up at between 9:00 AM and 10:30 PM........ Sometimes spending sleepless nights.

2. His food timings are at 11:00 AM - Breakfast or no Breakfast, 3:00 PM to 4:00 PM Lunch and dinner at 11:00 PM to 12:00 PM.

3. He was not doing any physical exercise for more than 10 years, not even walking 30 minutes a day for years.

4. He used to eat heavily because of long gaps between lunch and dinner and he used to make sure that Non-Veg is available most of the time, there were times when he did survey on city hotels, in the net to find delicious Non-Veg dishes. He was never interested in vegetable and healthier food.

5. Above all he was chain smoker from years.

6. His father passed away due to heart problems, and the doctors say the heart problems are usually genetic.

Once they identified the major block they have done immediately a procedure called angioplasty along with

2 Stints, mean they will insert a foreign body into the heart arteries and open the blocked area of arteries. He learnt from the doctors that 60% people will die before reaching the hospital, 20% people will die in the process of recovering from heart attack and only 20% will survive. In his case, he was very lucky to be part of the last 20%.

He was advised to have the physical exercise for minimum of 60 minutes on daily basis, to have food on time bound, consume food as less as possible, avoid the oily food, fried food, avoid smoking, sleep for minimum of 8 hours and keep practice the Yoga and more of medication.

So he urge you all to please avoid getting into this situation, it is in your hands to turn the situation upside down, by just planning / changing your life style, by following simple points above.

We have to learn from the Animals and birds, when they are sick they do not consume the food as fast as long as they are sick and give up only when they feel the signs of recovery. The ancient people have experimented the benefits of fasting and they have brought the customary practice in respective religion. The human organs need rest and by fasting it gets automatically rest. It is most unfortunate that human beings don't have as much control as animals. It is proven that in order to have active life, the food intake should be limited and in proportionate to the climatic and living conditions. In many cases food intake is ten times more than required and this cause the health disaster. It is well established fact that Fasting is constructive and starvation is destructive.

FIBROUS FOOD

Fibre plays a vital role in facilitating proper bower function. It's the indigestible part of vegetables, fruits and grains, which provides bulk to the food. Studies have shown that fibre rich diet helps in diabetes, in that it stabilizes blood sugar levels; lowers blood cholesterol levels and is associated with lower incidence of colon cancer, diverticulitis, constipation, hiatus hernia and hemorrhoids. Almost all the fibre comes from natural, unrefined, unprocessed food such as fruits, vegetables, legumes and whole—grain products. It is lost when food is processed and refined as in polished rice, white bread and maida which are low in fibre. Dairy products, eggs and meat have no dietary fibre, no matter how tough fibrous they may look. Consume lot of salad and fruits always before meals and never with or after. Salad is better than fruits.

Good Sources of Fibre

Fruits:

Apple, banana, berry orange, fig, pear dates, apricot, melon, mango, grapes, papaya, guava, jamun, raisin etc.,

Vegetables:

Peas, potato, sweet potato, beetroot, all green leafy vegetables, beans, carrot cabbage, ghiya, tori tinda, parwal, snake-gourd, etc.,

Legumes:

Dried whole pulses like rajma, whole moong, soya beans and all sprouts.

Grains:

Whole wheat, bajra, gram, ragi, jowar, barley, corn, unpolished rice and bran.

What are good for Good Health:

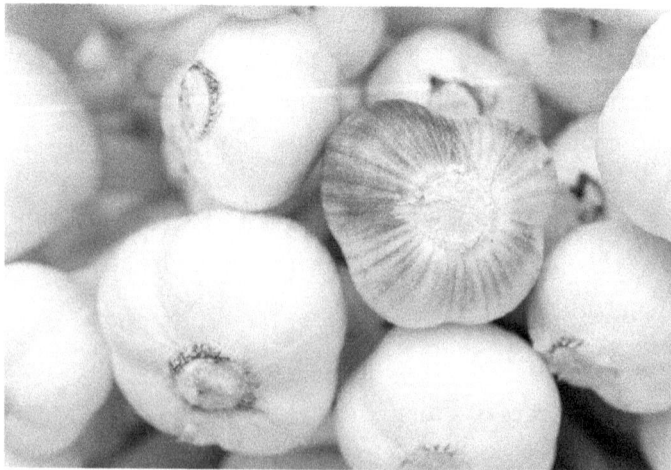

https://pixabay.com/en/aromatic-background-bulb-condiment-84691/

Garlic

Garlic is very good agent to reduce the blood pressure, blood cholesterol and triglycerides and also acts as antiseptic for killing all kinds of harmful bacteria/worms/germs etc., Research conducted all over the world reveals that Garlic is therefore good to have on regular basis if possible in every meal.

It is also a proven fact that cooked garlic is more recommended than the raw garlic. Cooking does not ruin its health giving properties, as in the case of others.

Raw garlic, if taken in excess quantity, in rare cases may cause irritation, burns and inflammation of the digestive tract, besides allergy, dermatitis, lethargy and dehydration. On the contrary well-cooked garlic is not irrigative and has no adverse effect.

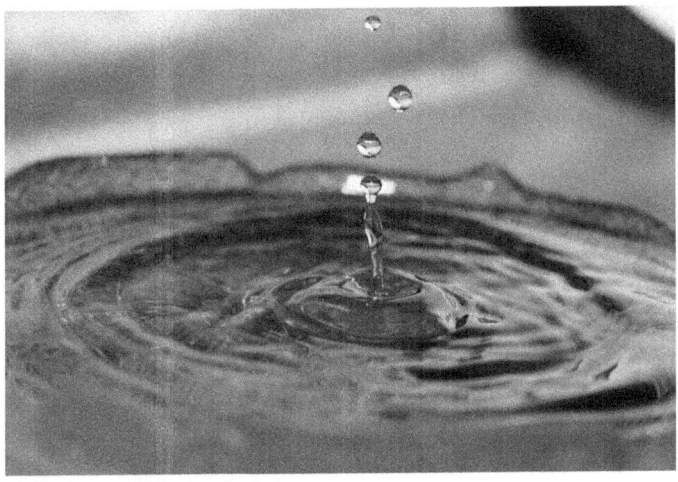

https://pixabay.com/en/waterdrop-water-drop-water-drop-2906/

Water

Water, which is the most essential and major component of body. The daily routine of the body depends on a turnover of about 40,000 glasses of water. Taking every now and then is good and especially in the morning hours and before going to bed. In the soft tissues-muscle, liver, kidney, the intestines-75 percent of the volume of the cells is water. The brain cell is said to be 85 percent water. The first impact of dehydration is felt by the brain cells; they are very sensitive to water loss from the body and their functions would be affected by even minute changes in their water contents. Dry mouth, thirsty are the indicators for the requirement of water. The body recycles this volume of water in 24 hours, but at the end it needs a minimum top up of about Twelve glasses in 24 hours. Tea, Coffee, cold drink and alcohol are not to be considered as water, these are in fact drying agents, and they force water out of the body. In the summer and humid periods and during continuous exercise, the human body needs more water for its cooling system (perspiration and sweating)- sometimes up to 10 to 15 or even more glasses a day.

RECOMMENDED WEIGHT CHART

Height	Men	Women
4.10ft(147.3cm)	---	48-52
4.11ft(150cm)	---	49-53
5ft (153cm)	56-58	50-54
5.1ft(155cm)	55-59	51-55
5.2ft(158cm)	56-60	53-56
5.3ft(160cm)	57-61	54-58
5.4ft(163cm)	59-63	56-59
5.5ft(165cm)	60-65	58-63
5.6ft(168cm)	62-66	58-63
5.7ft(170cm)	64-68	60-65
5.8ft(173cm)	65-70	62-66
5.9ft(175cm)	67-72	64-68
5.10ft(178cm)	69-74	65-70
5.11ft(180cm)	71-76	67-71
6ft(183cm)	73-78	68-71
6.1ft(185cm)	75-83	75-80
6.2ft(188cm)	77-83	---
6.3ft(190cm)	80-85	---

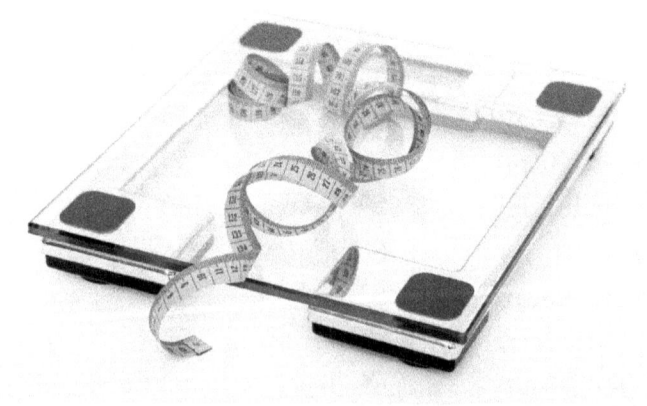

https://pixabay.com/en/scale-diet-fat-health-tape-weight-403585/

NORMAL / STANDARD LEVELS IN HUMAN BODY

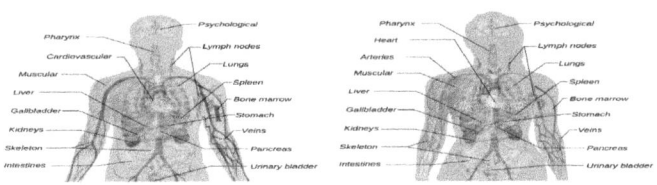

https://pixabay.com/en/
man-woman-schema-body-anatomy-144378/

TEST NAME	UNIT	NORMALRANGE
Serum creatinine	Mg%	0.5 – 1.4
Serum bilirubin, total	mg%	0.2 – 1.00
Serum Bilirubin, Conjugated	Mg%	0.2 – 0.4
Serum glutamic oxalacetic transaminase	U/L	5 – 40
Serum glutamic pyruvic transaminase	U/L	5 – 35
Serum alkaline phosphatase	IU/L	80-250 (Adults)/ Upto 600 Children)
Serum total proteins	gm%	6-8
Serum albumin	gm%	3.2 – 4.5
Serum globulin	gm%	2.3 – 3.5
Albumin/globulin ratio		2:1

TEST NAME	UNIT	NORMALRANGE
Hemoglobin	Gm%	14.0 – 18.0 (Male) 12.0 – 16.0 (Female)
Total White Cell Count	Cells/cumm	4000 – 11000
Different count polymorphs	%	60 – 70
Neutrophils	%	40 – 75%
Lymphocytes	%	20 – 30
Eosinophils	%	01 – 06
Monocyte	%	01 – 04
Total RBC Count	Millions/ cumm	3.2 – 5.0
Total platelet Count	Lacs/cumm	1.5 – 4.0
ESR	Mm/hr	0 – 07 (Male) 02 – 09 (Female)
PCV	%	40 – 54 (Male) 37 – 47 (Female)
MCV	fL	76 – 96
MCH	pg	32 – 36
MCHC	%	27 – 32
Random Blood Sugar	Mg/dl	100 – 160
Fasting Blood Sugar	Mg%	70 – 100
Blood Urea Nitrogen	Mg/dl	06 – 21
Blood Urea	Mg%	20 – 40
Basophils	%	0 – 5
Total lipids	Mg/dl	400 – 1000
Total triglycerides	mg/dl	90-150
Total Cholesterol	Mg/dl	150 – 200
High density lipoproteins (HDL)	Mg/dl	30 – 70
Low density lipoproteins (LDL)	Mg/dl	Up to 150

TEST NAME	UNIT	NORMALRANGE
Very low density lipoproteins (VLDL)	Mg/dl	25 – 40
Total cholesterol / HDL ratio		5: 1 (Males) 4.5: 1 (Females)
Uric acid	Mg/dl	3.4 – 8.0 (Male) 2.4 – 6.5
Calcium	Mg/dl	8.8 – 10.6
Phosphorous	Mg/dl	A. 2.7 – 4.5 C. 4.0 – 7.0
Total proteins	Gm/dl	6.0 – 8.0
Aspartate Amino Transferase (SGOT)	IU/L	0 – 37 (Male) 0 – 31 (Female)
Alanine Amino Transferase (SGPT)	IU/L	0 – 40 (Male) 0-31 (Female)
Alkaline phosphatase (ALP)	U/L	A. 39 - 130 C. 70 – 550
Gamma GT	U/L	10 – 87 (Male) 8 – 39 (Female)
Red cell count	Mill/cu mm	4.5 – 6.5 3.8 – 5.8

FOOD CALORIES LIST

BREADS & CEREALS	Portion size *	per 100 grams (3.5 oz)	energy content
Bagel (1 average)	140 cals (45g)	310 cals	Medium
Biscuit digestives	86 cals (per biscuit)	480 cals	High
Jaffa cake	48 cals (per biscuit)	370 cals	Med-High
Bread white (thick slice)	96 cals (1 slice 40g)	240 cals	Medium
Bread wholemeal (thick)	88 cals (1 slice 40g)	220 cals	Low-med
Chapatis	250 cals	300 cals	Medium
Cornflakes	130 cals (35g)	370 cals	Med-High
Crackerbread	17 cals per slice	325 cals	Low Calories
Cream crackers	35 cals (per cracker)	440 cals	Low / portion
Crumpets	93 cals (per crumpet)	198 cals	Low-Med
Flapjacks basic fruit mix	320 cals	500 cals	High
Macaroni (boiled)	238 cals (250g)	95 cals	Low calorie
Muesli	195 cals (50g)	390 cals	Med-high

Naan bread (normal)	300 cals (small plate size)	320 cals	Medium
Noodles (boiled)	175 cals (250g)	70 cals	Low calorie
Pasta (normal boiled)	330 cals (300g)	110 cals	Low calorie
Pasta (wholemeal boiled)	315 cals (300g)	105 cals	<u>Low calorie</u>
Porridge oats (with water)	193 cals (350g)	55 cals	Low calorie
Potatoes** (boiled)	210 cals (300g)	70 cals	Low calorie
Potatoes** (roast)	420 cals (300g)	140 cals	Medium
Rice (white boiled)	420 cals (300g)	140 cals	<u>Low calorie</u>
Rice (egg-fried)	500 cals	200 cals	High in portion
Rice (Brown)	405 cals (300g)	135 cals	Low calorie
Rice cakes	28 Cals = 1 slice	373 Cals	Medium
Ryvita Multi grain	37 Cals per slice	331 Cals	Medium
Ryvita + seed & Oats	180 Cals 4 slices	362 Cals	Medium
Spaghetti (boiled)	303 cals (300g)	101 cals	Low calorie

HEALTH IS THE ONLY REAL WEALTH

"A fit, healthy body—that is the best statement"

"Let food be thy medicine and medicine be thy food."

"We are healthy only to the extent that our ideas are humane."

"Healthy citizens are the greatest asset any country can have."

"Money cannot buy health, but I'd settle for a diamond-studded wheelchair."

"The First wealth is health."

"I am not my body. My body is nothing without me."

"Eat healthily, sleep well, breathe deeply, move harmoniously."

"Respect your body. Eat well. Dance forever."

"When health is absent, wisdom cannot reveal itself, art cannot manifest, strength cannot fight, wealth becomes useless, and intelligence cannot be applied."

"When wealth is lost, nothing is lost and when Health is lost, everything is lost."

"I could never kill myself. I approve of suicide if you have horrible health. Otherwise it's the ultimate hissy fit."

"True discipline is really just self-remembering; no forcing or fighting is necessary."

"Each patient carries his own doctor inside him."

"Sunshine, water, rest, fresh air, Exercise and diet, is must for good health."

"1 billion people in the world are chronically hungry. 1 billion people are overweight."

"No disease that can be treated by diet should be treated with any other means."

"Anger's like a battery that leaks acid right out of me and it starts from the heart 'til it reaches my outer me"

"Will is a skill." Have a will to keep your body fit and healthy, you can do any type of work.

"It is easier to change a man's religion than to change his diet."

"Eating crappy food isn't a reward -- it's a punishment."

"To wish a healthy man to die is the wish from a mind of sickness. To wish an ailing man to die is the wish of the ambitious."

"May your heart be lighter today?"

"The body is wiser than its inhabitants. The body is the soul. The body is god's messenger."

"Health makes good propaganda."

"Health nuts are going to feel stupid someday, lying in hospitals dying of nothing..."

"Health isn't about being "perfect" with food or exercise or herbs. Health is about balancing those things with your desires."

"It's true that laughter really is cheap medicine. It's a prescription anyone can afford. And best of all, you can fill it right now."

"Meditation is the ultimate mobile device; you can use it anywhere, anytime, unobtrusively."

"Sorry, there's no magic bullet. You got to eat healthy and live healthy to be healthy and look healthy."

"If your arteries are good, eat more ice cream. If they are bad, drink more red wine."

"Time and time again, throughout the history of medical practice, what was once considered as "scientific" eventually becomes regarded as "bad practice"."

"I didn't want to upset my loved ones, but I couldn't carry this alone."

"Health is the greatest possession. Contentment is the greatest treasure. Confidence is the greatest friend."

"A little chocolate a day keeps the doctor at bay"

"If you don't take care of this the most magnificent machine that you will ever be given...where are you going to live?"

"Have good health and Live Life Fully & Abundantly."

"The most poetical thing in the world is not being sick."

"About eighty percent of the food on shelves of supermarkets today didn't exist 100 years ago."

"You spend your TIME to make a DIME. You lose your HEALTH to make your WEALTH, but at the end it is FUNNY because you leave back all your MONEY."

"You are what you eat. What would YOU like to be?"

"Tell me what you eat and I will tell you who you are."

"There is no illness that is not exacerbated by stress."

"You only get one body; it is the temple of your soul. Even God is willing to dwell there. If you truly treat your body like a temple, it will serve you well for decades. If you abuse it you must be prepared for poor health and a lack of energy."

"Healthy people have a natural skill of avoiding feverish eyes."

"Managing perfect body weight is not a complicated rocket science."

"Never take today for granted, tomorrow might never come."

"Humor and Health, are the staples of wealth."

"Walk 1 and Drink 8. Walk 1 km and drink 8 cups of water every day."

"There are many things to resist, but disease is not one of them."

"Not only a man without hand, is handicapped but also a man without health."

"Stop taking identity in illness and start taking identity in wellness"

"The greatest wealth is well-being."

"Your health is a testament to your life. The better your quality of health, in all likelihood the longer your life."

"Your life, your health and your weight are 80% due to what you eat, and 20% due to activity level."

"Your body is an integral part of your intuition."

"Health is the main capital one possesses and better administer it intelligently."

"Health is the greatest strength."

"God can cure any illness."

"Dancing every night enhances a positive energy."

"Love your body. Exercise for 10-15 minutes daily."

"Good health is a holy blessing."

"Motivation is soothing medicine for the soul."

"Make time daily for your well-being."

"The grace of joyful living gives strength to the bones."

"Physical activity promotes high productivity."

HEALTH IS EVERYTHING, PRESERVE GOOD HEALTH AT ANY COST.

BRIEF PROFILE OF CA. DR. VISHNU BHARATH AS

PRESENT:

- Practicing Sr. Chartered Accountant from past 42 years
- Vice President of APS Education Trust,(80 years of repute)
- Chairman – PHF Co., (P) Ltd-Transit Living Service Apartments
- Executive President – Karnataka Federation of United Nations UNESCO
- Director – CANFINA Financial Services, Subsidiary of Canara Bank.
- Chairman –RV Integrated PU College
- Chairman – Education committee of FKCCI
- President – Vasavi Vedha Nidhi Trust, Sancrit school.
- Trustee – Welfare Trust of GMR Infra.
- Trustee – RSS Trust, RV Institutions, Bangalore (Institution of 75 years)
- Member – Fiscal Laws Committee (FICCI), New Delhi

PAST: EXPERIENCE:

- Chairman – Southern India Regional Council of Institute of Chartered Accountants of India. Recipient of Best Region award of ICAI
- President – Karnataka State Chartered Accountants Association
- Chairman – Bangalore Branch of SIRC of ICAI. Received
- Best Branch award of ICAI.
- Managing Committee Member of FKCCI.

- President – Vasavi CA Charitable Trust.
- Chairman – NMKRV Degree College.
- Income tax practice & Bank Audit from past 42 years.
- Principal Statutory Auditor for Vysya Bank Ltd.,
- Principal Tax Auditor for Entire Canara Bank for three years.
- Adviser to Vijaya Bank.
- Branch Audits of State Bank of Mysore, State Bank of Travancore, Syndicate Bank,& Canara Bank.
- Tax consultant for The Vysya Bank Ltd., for over three decades.

AWARDS:

- HONORABLE DOCTRATE for Social Service and contribution to Society received from Mangalore University.
- HONORARY PROFESSORSHIP for Communication skills by Tumkur University.
- RASHTREEYA UDYOG, VIKAS JYOTHI Award. VASAVI SIRI Award, KANNADA SIRI,

AUTHORED:

- AUTHORED 24 BOOKS, "LIFE IS LIKE A JOURNEY ON A TRAIN" & "HEALTH IS WEALTH AND IT IS TAX FREE" are published by Penguin Co., international publisher and made it available in 158 countries.
- PERSONAL GUIDE TO INCOME TAX Published by FKCCI.
- A WOMANS WORLD – Released by Governor of Karnataka.
- A MAN'S WORLD – All about how to achieve success
- KNOW MORE – Knowledge is Strength
- ARYA VYSYA BOOK- All about Arya Vysya's
- "HEALTH IS WALTH AND IT IS TAX FREE" Tips for good health.
- "LIFE IS PRECIOUS" Importance of Human life.

- "BANK UPON YOUR BANK" Sponsored by FKCCI.
- "VARIETY IS SPICE IN LIFE" Short stories.
- "FESTIVALS OF INDIA" All about Indian Festivals. Spon by PJH Ltd.,
- "I LOVE MY INDIA" Sponsored by Canara Bank.
- "WORDS OF WISDOM" Sponsored by ITC Ltd.,
- "FAILURE IS STEPPING STONE FOR SUCCESS" spon by GMR Infra
- "LIFE, FRIENDSHIP & HAPPINESS" sponsored by GMR Infra Ltd.,
- "ADINARAYANA MAHIME" of SLAS Charitable Trust.
- "V CAT REFERENCER" A guide for Business man Spon by VCAT
- "GOD THE ALMIGHTY" Sponsored by Canara Bank.
- "LIFE IS A LIKE A JOURNEY ON A TRAIN"- God is Travel Agent.
- "KILL THE ILL WITH OUT THE PILL – HERBAL REMEDIES"
- "SMILE & SMILE ALL THE WAY – Spon by M/s Advaith Hyundai.
- "CENTURIAN SMT. NARMADABAI." Spon By APS Edu Trust.
- "PAST, PRESENT & FUTURE" Sponsored by M/s Abaran Jewellers.
- "LIVE LIFE BEFORE YOU LEAVE LIFE" By M/s Tallam Apperals.
- "FLIP FLOP INDIA" Sponsored by Can Fin Homes Ltd.,

OTHERS:
- Toured all over the world & Member of Red Cross Society
- Given Interview in AIR and Doordarshan – Public Cause
- Has keen interest in Farming and Agriculture
- Good Sportsman and Regular Swimmer &Yoga enthusiast

Address: No. 7/8, 2nd Floor, Shoukath Building, SJP Road, Bangalore -2.
Residence: No. 450, 7th Main, 4th Block, Jayanagar, Bangalore 11.
Phone Nos.42104220 & Mobile: 98807 01701& 99800 77078
Email: vishnubharathco@gmail.com,
Web: www.vishnubharath.com

www.ingramcontent.com/pod-product-compliance
Lightning Source LLC
Chambersburg PA
CBHW070946200526
45161CB00001BA/1